Natural Remedies for Bites and Stings

Peter Bigfoot

Illustrations by
Kentree Speirs

Reevis Mountain School of Self-Reliance
7448 S. J-B Ranch Rd.
Roosevelt, AZ 85545
www.reevismountain.org
info@reevismountain.org

© Copyright 1990, 2010 by Peter Bigfoot. All rights reserved.

Revised July 2010

ISBN 978-0-9824091-1-4 / 0-9824091-1-7

Natural Remedies for Bites and Stings

Peter Bigfoot

Illustrations by
Kentree Speirs

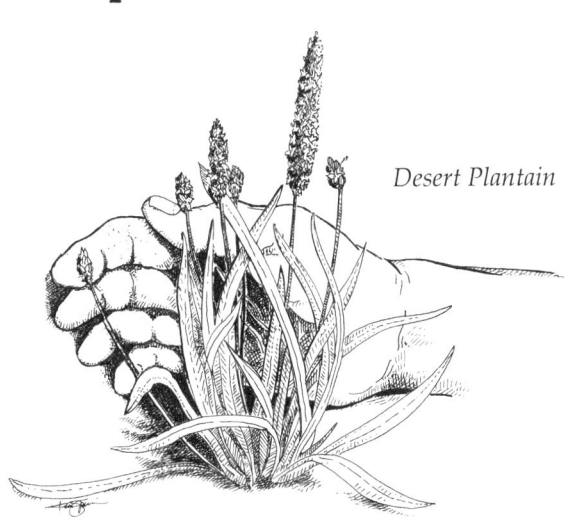

Desert Plantain

Contents

Introduction   1
General Word of Caution   5
Snake Bites   7
    Remedies   8
Spider Bites   17
    Remedies   21
Scorpion Stings   25
    Remedies   33
Bee, Ant, and Wasp Stings   37
    Remedies   39
    Allergic Reaction (Anaphylactic Shock)   47
Other Insects   49
    Mosquitoes, Gnats, and Flies   49
    Scabies   49
    Lice   51
    Fleas and Ticks   51
    Chiggers   53
    Kissing Bugs, Cone Nose Beetles, Hualapai Tigers   55
    Blister Beetles   55
Gila Monsters   57
Other Animal Bites   57
    Remedies   57
Rabid Animal Bites   59
    Remedies   61
Poison Ivy   63
How to Make the Remedies   67
    Poultices   67
    Fomentations   73
    Herb Teas   75
    Canaigre Root Juice   77
    Urine Therapy   77
Reevis Mountain School of Self-Reliance   79

Index of Plants

Alder tree (*Alnus* spp.)   65
Algerita (*Mahonia fremontii*)   59
Ash tree (*Fraxinus* spp.; Common Ash *F. excelsior*)   15, 61
Aspen tree (*Populus tremuloides*)   14, **30**, 33, 43, 77
Barrel cactus (*Ferocactus wislizenil*)   **6**, 9, 14, 71, 73
Bistort (*Persicaria bistorta*)   15
Black Cohosh (*Actaea racemosa, Cimicifuga racemosa*)   **10**, 11, 13, 23, 27, 35, 39, 45, 47
Camphor weed (*Heterotheca grandiflora*)   49, 53, **76**, **78**
Canaigre (*Rumex hymenosepalus*)   55, 57, **58**, 59, 61, 77
Castor (*Ricinus communis*)   **34**, 35
Catnip (*Nepeta cataria*)   47
Chamomile (*Matricaria recutita*)   47
Chaparral (*Larrea divaricata, L. tridentata*)   19, 21, 22, 23, **28**, 35, 45, 47, 49, 51, 53, 59
Chickweed (*Stellaria* spp.)   43, **46**
Comfrey (*Symphytum officinale*)   19
Cottonwood tree (*Populus fremontii*)   14, 27, **31**, 33, 43, 47
Cypress tree (*Cupressus sempervirens*)   59, 61
Datura (*Datura meteloides*)   21, 23, **48**, 49, 67
Desert Lavender (*Hyptis emoryi*)   21, 22, 23, **40**, 41
Desert Plantain (*Plantago insularis*)   **title page**, 11, 13, 21, 23, 35, 43, 45, 49, 51, 55
Desert Tobacco (*Nicotiana trigonophylla*)   14, **38**, 41, 45, 55
Desert Willow (*Chilopsis linearis*)   51, **52**, 53, 57, 61
Echinacea (*Echinacea angustifolia, E. purpurea, E. pallida, Brauneria angustifolia*)   11, **12**, 13, 15, 23, 45, 47, 51, 53, 55, 59, 61, 65
English Lavender (*Lavandula* spp.)   65
Ephedra (*Ephedra sinica*)   **44**, 47

Fennel (*Foeniculum officinale, F. vulgare*)   14, 15, 47
Four Wing Salt Bush (*Atriplex canescens*)   41, 43, **74**
Goldenseal (*Hydrastis canadensis*)   59
Green Gentian (*Swertia radiata, Frasera speciosa*)   49, **50**, 51, 61
Hedgehog cactus (*Mammillaria* spp.)   **8**, 14, 23, 41, 71
Jewel Weed (*Impatiens pallida, I. capensis*)   65
Lambsquarter (*Chenopodium berlandieri*)   65
Lanceleaf Plantain (*Plantago lanceolata*)   65
Lemonade bush (*Rhus trilobata*)   71
Motherwort (*Leonurus cardiaca*)   47
Oak tree (*Quercus* spp.)   30, 49, 65, 77
Oshá (*Ligusticum porteri*)   59, 61
Papaya (*Carica papaya*)   41
Pasture Bindweed (*Convolvulus arvensis*)   21
Poison Ivy (*Toxicodendron radicans*)   2, **62**, 63, 65
Prickly Pear cactus (*Opuntia polyacantha basilaris*)   **4**, 9, 21, 23, 25, 27, 33, 41, 47, 51, 55, 66, 68, 69, 70
Purslane (*Portulaca oleracea*)   33, **42**, 43, 55
Sand Spurge (*Euphorbia exserta*)   14, 41, **72**, 73
Sycamore tree (*Planatus wrightii*)   65
Tree Tobacco (*Nicotiana glauca*)   41
Turpentine Brush (*Haplopappus laricifolius*)   43
Valerian (*Valeriana officinalis, V. arizonica, V. edulis*)   47, **60**
Walnut tree (*Juglans nigra, J. major*)   15, 21, 23, 49, 51, **56**, 59, 61, 65
Water Pepper (*Polygonum punctatum*)   53
Western Mugwort (*Artemisia vulgaris, A. ludoviciana*)   29, 30, **32**, 33, 35, 45, 47, 49, 53, 63, 65
Wild Grape (*Vitis arizonica*)   15, **64**, 65
Wild Iris (*Iris* spp.)   61
Yarrow (*Achillea lanulosa, A. millefolium*)   49
Yellow Dock (*Rumex crispus*)   59, 61
Yerba Santa (*Eriodictyon glutinosum*)   65

Introduction

One day in 1948, when I was six years old, I made the mistake of urinating into a yellow jacket hive and received 13 stings. Ever since that day, I have been interested in simple natural remedies for venomous bites and stings.

In 1980 I helped to found and create a homestead in the Superstition Wilderness of Arizona, and I still live here, with my wife and a changing group of interns and students. We enjoy the great beauty and diversity of geology and vegetation, but as we and our neighbors know, everything in the desert will "stick you, sting you, bite you, or burn you."

In our wilderness home we live closely with rattlesnakes, scorpions, brown recluse and black widow spiders, gnats, chiggers, bees, wasps, blister beetles, kissing bugs, ants, skunks, fox, and bears. We have also had some — fortunately rare — experience with fleas, ticks, lice, scabies, rabies, and Poison Ivy.

That we have found simple, effective, natural remedies for the bites and stings that our wild neighbors sometimes inflict on us helps us to be much more confident and comfortable about living in the back country. For example, knowing how to remedy a snake bite with the use of local wild plants allays much of the fear associated with being around snakes, and so on.

We read in the newspaper once of a man from Mesa, Arizona, who was bitten by a brown recluse spider. Medical treatment cost him $60,000 and the loss of his hand. From our experience with the remedies found in this book, a serious spider bite would be no more than a minor inconvenience.

It has been brought to our attention that we have something of great value and importance to share.

The information in this book is organized by animal

so that you can find the remedies quickly in the event of a bite or sting. I have included remedies for Poison Ivy, as it is a common source of discomfort in the wilderness and, being natural, also has simple natural remedies that will be found nearby. A section at the end of the book describes how to make the remedies. These are the simple and effective remedies that we use on a regular and ongoing basis. They work very well for us and offer the same to you.

For each critter you might get tangled up with, we offer several remedies so that you can have options to choose from—not that you have to use them all at once. It is advisable to read this book *before* the remedy is needed so you will be prepared when an emergency occurs.

It is important to note that the remedies mentioned herein are by no measure the only ones that could be used. These are just a starting point. You may find many more once you start looking. I want you to realize that Nature has lots of remedies, and you've got the power. Make use of both.

Peter Bigfoot

DISCLAIMER

This book is intended to share information about what has worked for us. We make no claims or guarantees about what it can do for you. If you use these methods, you must use them at your own risk.

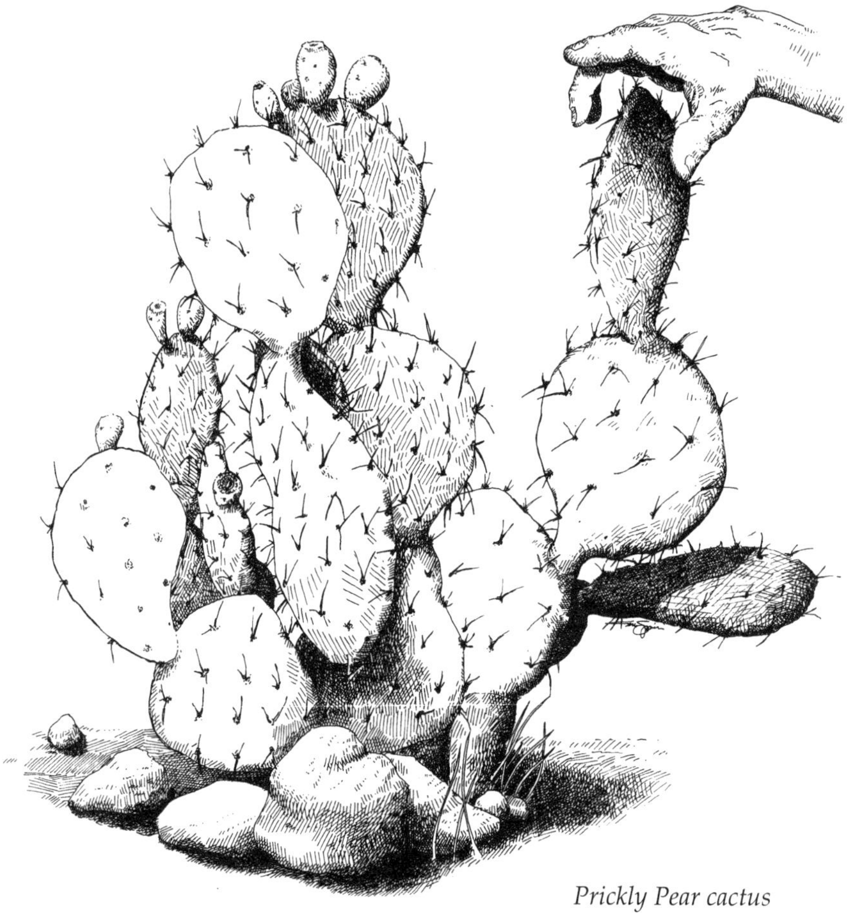

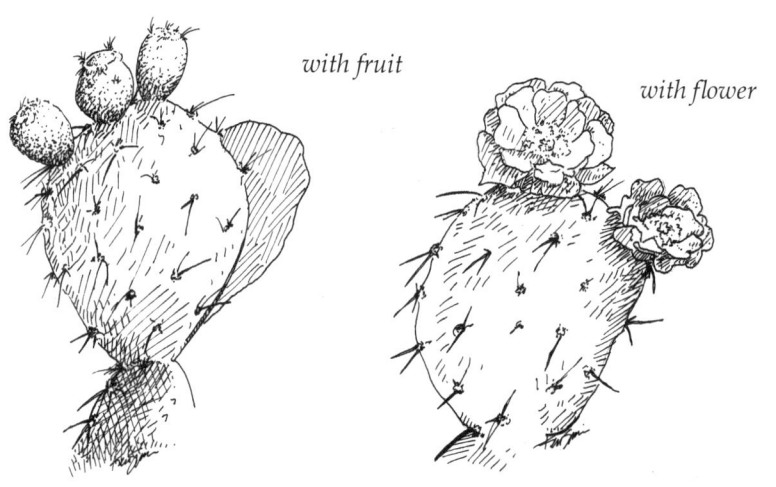

Prickly Pear cactus

with fruit

with flower

General Word of Caution

Do not rub, scratch, or massage venomous bites and stings. Do not apply any heat. All of these will make the condition much worse. We don't put any faith in a conventional snake bite kit.

For stings received while in the ocean (e.g., sting rays), we have heard it is best to apply heat, not cold.

For bites and stings, as with any injury, do not procrastinate about treatment. The sooner you get on it, the less damage will be done and the quicker you will heal.

Venomous bites and stings are natural occurrences, and the remedies are often found in nature, most always in the area where the event occurs.

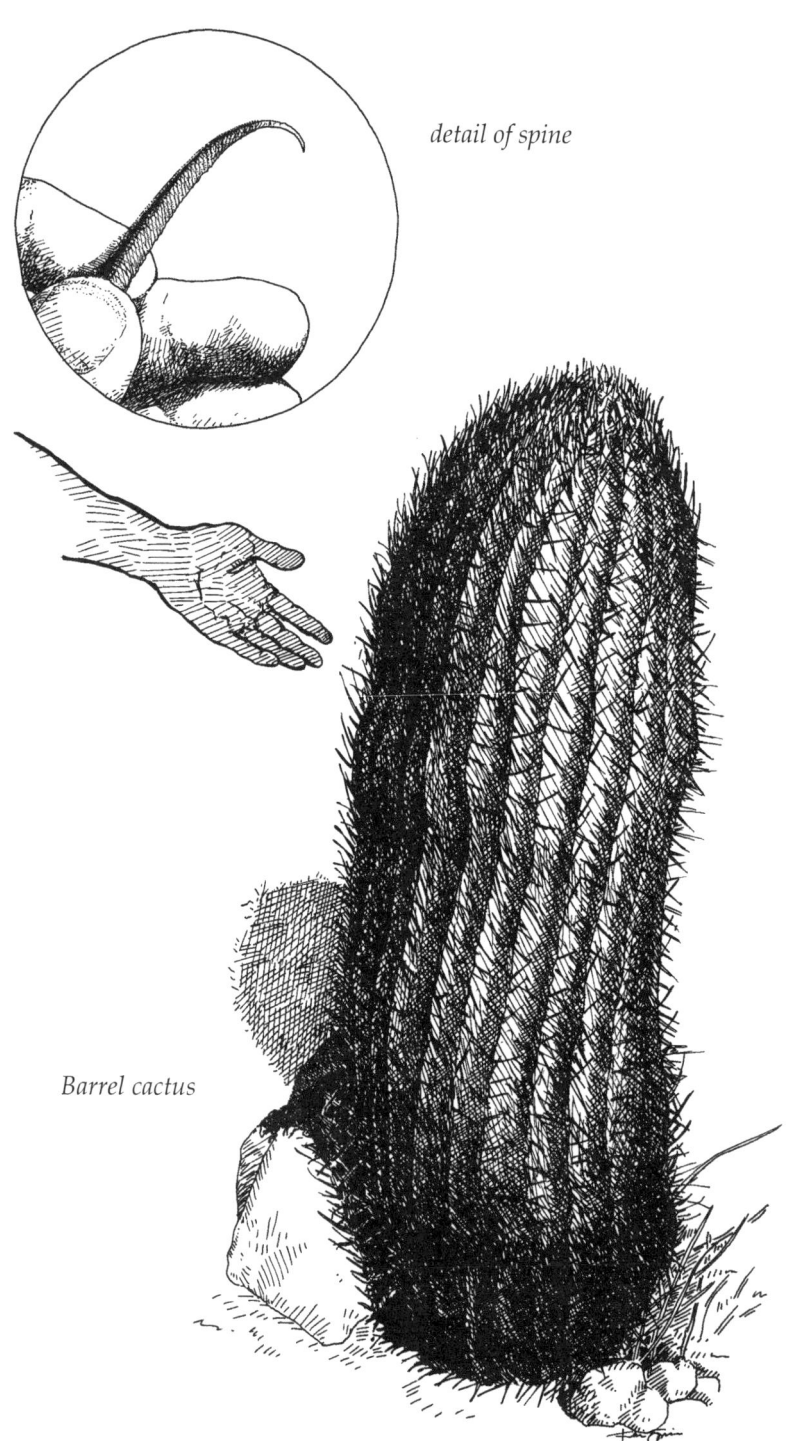

detail of spine

Barrel cactus

Snake Bites

If you see a rattlesnake, calmly move away. Rattlesnakes do not chase people—they only try to protect themselves from getting stepped on. There is no need to kill a rattlesnake unless you need something to eat.

Personally, I have been around many rattlesnakes and have never been bitten. We have observed that the rattlesnakes seem to respond to our thoughts, attitude, and intent. If they feel safe they are less likely to bite.

When a two-legged, five-foot-plus monster comes too close for his comfort, a male rattlesnake will rattle more readily and be more likely to defend himself than the more timid female. She will most likely lay quietly still and depend on her camouflage to protect her. If she gets stepped on, she may bite to get away.

I have talked with several people who have been bitten by rattlesnakes, and they say that, unlike bee stings, rattlesnake bites seldom hurt at first. At first, the bite feels like you were slapped with a twig. About 15 minutes to a half hour later swelling begins and the pain increases, and increases, and increases. The bite may feel different for different varieties of snakes.

Even though our experience has mostly been with rattlesnakes, I feel that most of these remedies will be good for other varieties of snakes as well.

Remedies

If I were bit by a rattlesnake, the first thing I would do would be to stay calm. Then I would work quickly. Each moment is precious—the faster the remedies are applied, the quicker the healing.

There is something about working the muscles that makes the bite get worse. It may be the extra circulation and body heat generated that compound the injury. Venom is a hot energy; keep mentally and physically cool so as not to increase that heat.

The first thing to do is whatever can be done most quickly: either drink some of the suggested tea or apply a poultice. If you have a choice, apply the poultice first and then drink the tea. Follow the instructions for the specific type of poultice, and drink the suggested tea each hour or as needed. Rest until healed.

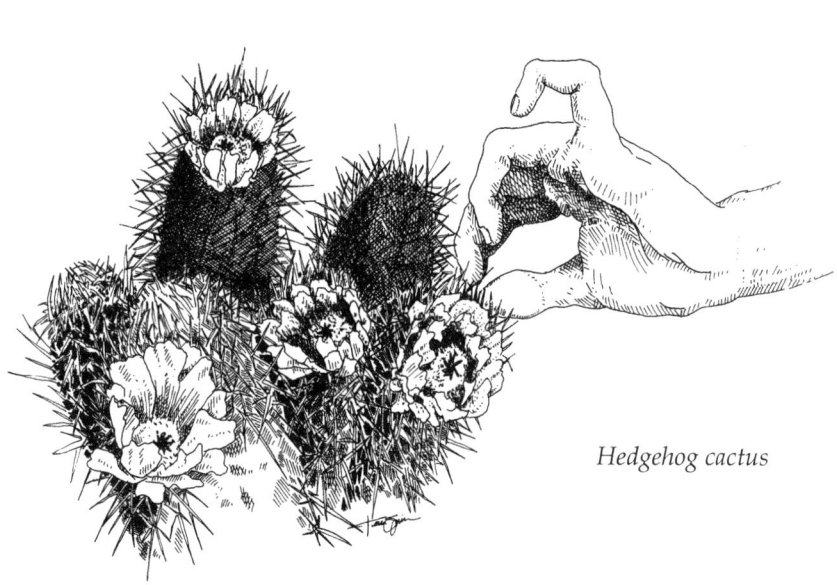

Hedgehog cactus

Poultices & Fomentations

Bites and stings often create a lot of localized heat and swelling. Changing the poultice when it begins to feel hot seems to hasten the healing process.

When applying poultices over snake bites, cover at least a six-inch diameter area around the bite. Whenever the poultice feels that it has become saturated with heat or dried out, apply a fresh poultice. Continue applying poultices until healed, one to three days.

Barrel Cactus Poultice: Apply a large poultice (one pint to one quart) of mashed Barrel cactus flesh to the bite site, or submerge the bitten area (as for the hand) in a bowl of mashed Barrel cactus flesh.

Prickly Pear Cactus Poultice: Apply a large Prickly Pear cactus pad to the bite site. Change the pad every hour until healed.

One of my students told me about a time when he was out in the desert and began to pick up a rock off the ground. A rattlesnake was under a little Bursage bush and it struck out and bit him on the wrist.

He was out there all alone and believed, as I do, that most likely there would be a natural remedy nearby. After centering himself in a meditative mood to receive guidance, he remembered the Prickly Pear cactus. He rubbed the spines off a pad with a rough stone, cut the cactus pad open, and applied it to the bite.

He said he had felt a deadly energy moving up his arm. It had gotten to his armpit and begun to swell the glands there. After applying the cactus pad he could feel the energy retracting, and in a few hours it had left his hand.

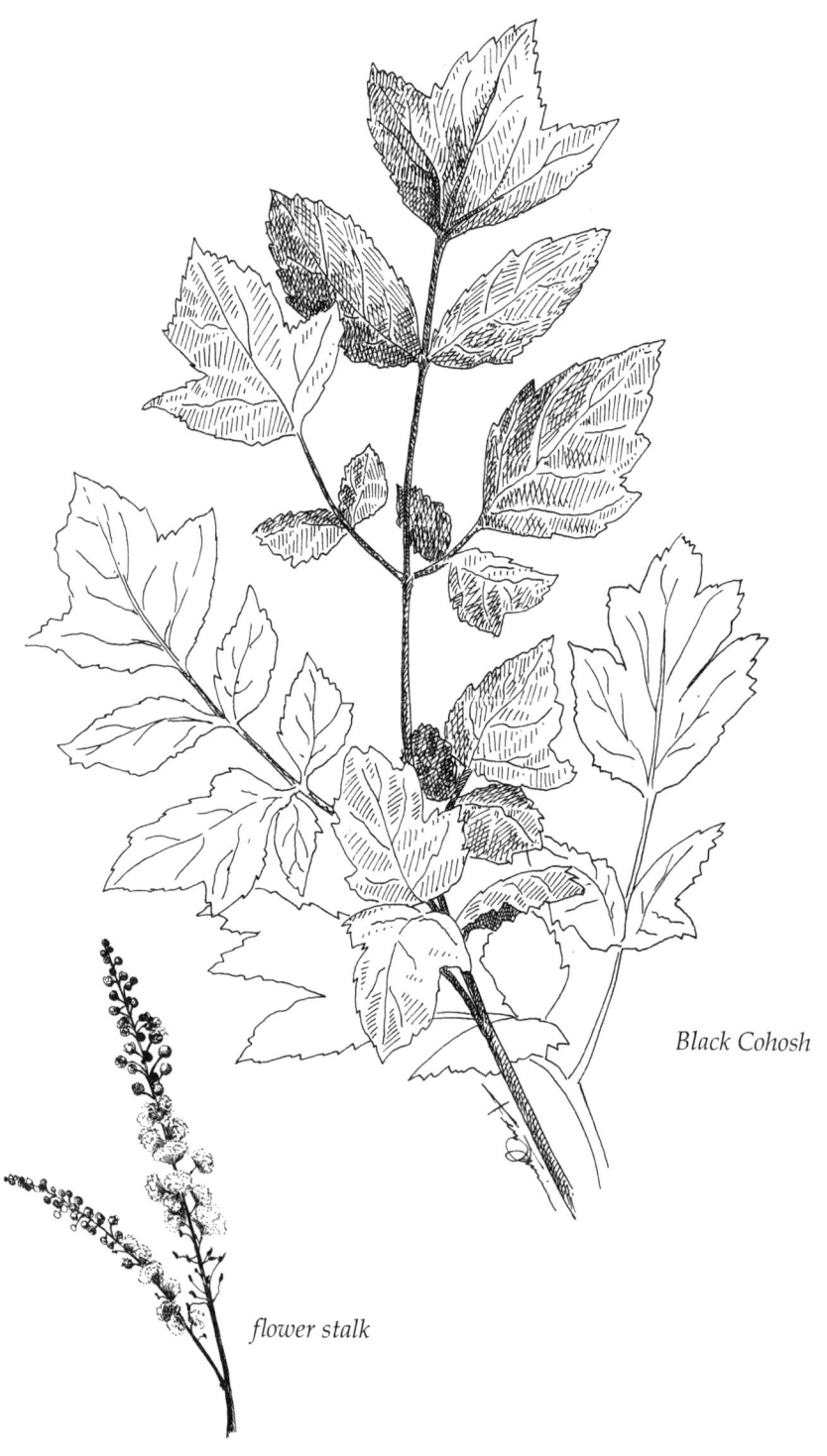

A friend's son, age about 12, was bitten on his finger by a sidewinder rattlesnake. At first, the boy and his father didn't think much of it because it didn't hurt and the snake was so small. An hour later the swelling and pain were becoming intense.

They were from Phoenix but were on a two-week camping trip to Colorado, so they were far away from home. The father remembered about Black Cohosh, and happened to have some along. The boy began drinking Black Cohosh tea, and it was effective. In a day or two the bite was 95% healed and the boy was rapidly on the mend.

Then they got themselves talked into taking the boy to a hospital in Durango. In only 24 hours the boy had relapsed and become extremely ill. The parents had enough of that and removed the boy from the hospital, but first they had to pay $1,400! They finally got their son well again with herbs. It took nearly a month to undo the damage from whatever was done in the hospital.

Desert Plantain Poultice: Apply a large poultice of fresh bruised plants or the dried and powdered herb reconstituted with water. We use the entire plant.

Black Cohosh Root Fomentation: Apply a thick mass of cotton cloth (wadded or folded) over the wound area, saturated with a strong, cool solution of the tea. Keep the cloth saturated and do not let it dry out. If you don't have cloth available, use dirt and make a mud poultice.

Clay and Echinacea Root: We heard about this remedy from someone who used it with favorable results. Moisten the desired amount of dry clay powder with strong tea or tincture of Echinacea root and apply over the wound. Keep the clay saturated; do not let it dry out.

Echinacea Root Fomentation: Use the same method as for Black Cohosh root above. Use fresh tea of dried root or a tincture of the root. I like the tincture better, if available.

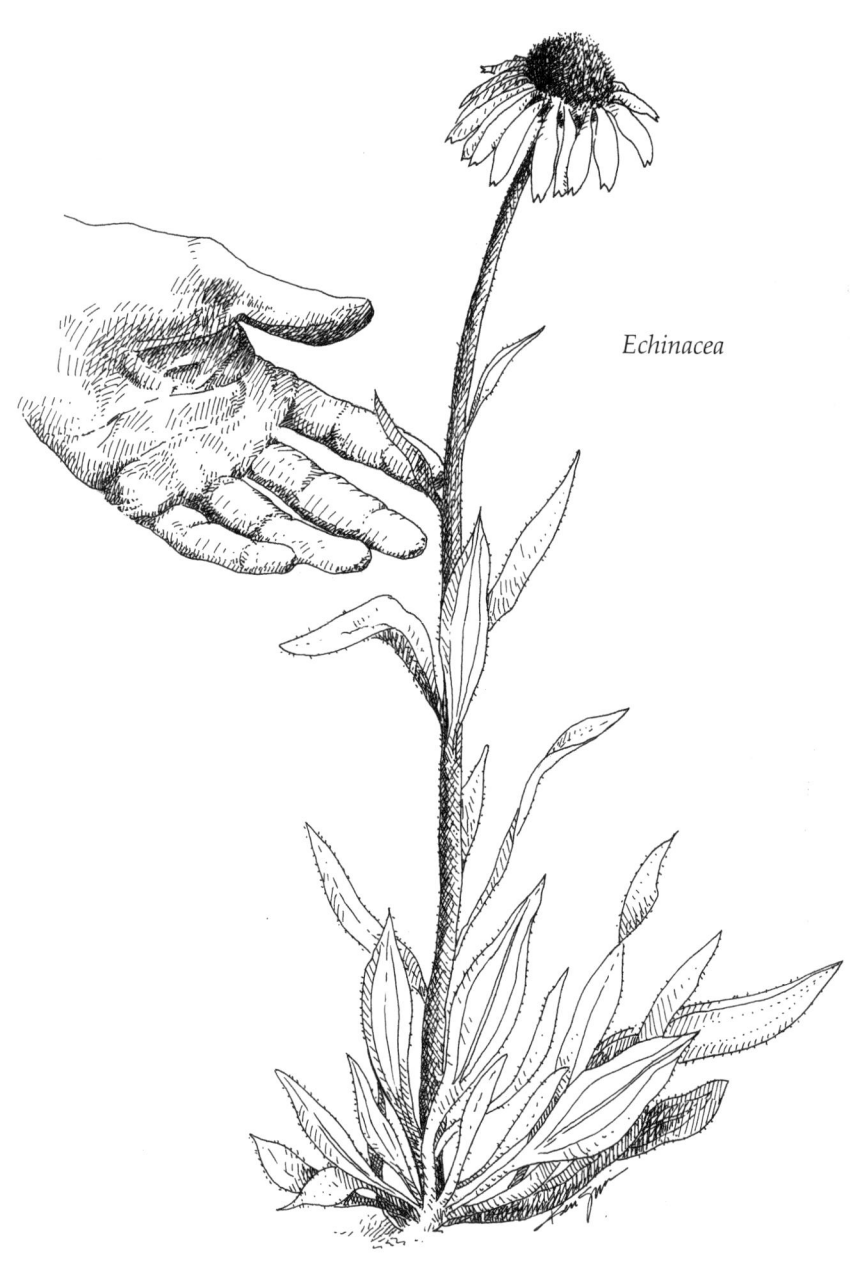

Herb Teas

Black Cohosh Root: Every hour or so, as needed, drink one cup of tea, brewed to taste. Pay attention to how the tea feels to you – you may wish to drink more or less accordingly. It is possible to overdo on Black Cohosh.

Echinacea Root: This is one of our most trusted remedies. Drink tea made from the dried root or root tincture, one cup every so often as needed.

Desert Plantain Leaf: Every hour, drink a cup or more brewed to taste.

The above remedies are the ones we trust the most. The following remedies are ones that we have heard work. We feel they would be worth a try if you do not have the above available.

Our farm cat named Bogart got bitten in the face by a rattlesnake. He came in the house with his head swollen up like a pumpkin. I squirted about three droppers full of Echinacea tincture, full strength, down his throat and rubbed some Echinacea tincture into his fur around the bite area. The cat began to foam and froth from his mouth, like a bubbling-over pop bottle, for several minutes. About two hours later the swelling was nearly gone, and by the next day he was back to normal.

Since the experience with Bogart, our cat friends Ben and Miriam also have been bitten. We gave them Echinacea tincture diluted with water, a half teaspoon of tincture to a tablespoon of water. We gave about two quarter-ounce doses with the dropper that comes in the bottle. Then we gently rubbed the full-strength tincture on their fur in the bite area.

The diluted tincture did not make the cats foam and froth, and they recovered quickly.

Additional Poultices/Fomentations

Fresh liver, raw shredded potato, ice, Hedgehog cactus, Cottonwood or Aspen tree leaves (fresh), tobacco (especially fresh green Desert Tobacco), mud (wet soil), fomentation of your own urine, the milky sap from fresh Sand Spurge stems, crushed Fennel seed, Adolf's Meat Tenderizer.

As a fomentation, the Bee/Insect Sting Remedy that we make seems to be good for a wide variety of bites and stings, but it has not been tried on snake bites yet.

One of my students told me a friend of his had been bitten by a rattlesnake two days before. I had made some Barrel cactus remedy (see page 71) ten days earlier and was eager to try it out.

The friend had been running a trail in South Mountain Park in Phoenix when he stepped on the snake, and it bit his ankle. He felt no pain, and so thought maybe he had a "dry bite," but figured he'd best get it checked out by a doctor. He walked a half mile back to his car and drove to a hospital. By this time the pain and swelling were getting intense.

The hospital folks gave him some antibiotics but said that because of his body chemistry the anti-venom would do more harm than good. Four hours later, as he was leaving the hospital, he could barely function.

The next day the leg was swollen and a dark blue-purple color — nearly black — and extremely painful. His doctor told him that cutting the leg off would be better than having it rot off, which he felt was imminent.

Early on the third day my student applied a one-pint poultice of the Barrel cactus remedy. Within 15 minutes the friend felt some relief. They left the poultice on for about 36 hours. The third day after they put the poultice on, this fellow went out for a long day hike to celebrate his newly healed leg. It was a miraculous recovery!

Additional Herb Teas

Wild Grape leaf, Walnut tree bark, Ash tree root bark, Bistort root, Fennel seed.

Urine

Urine is the most popular remedy used in India for snake bites. It is believed that a person's urine becomes a homeopathic remedy after venom enters the blood. I do not have any firsthand experience with this remedy. At least it's cheap. See page 77.

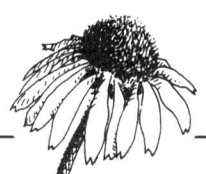

After observing, so many times, how easily and how well the Echinacea treatment has worked, I feel that Echinacea is our primary choice for snake bites.

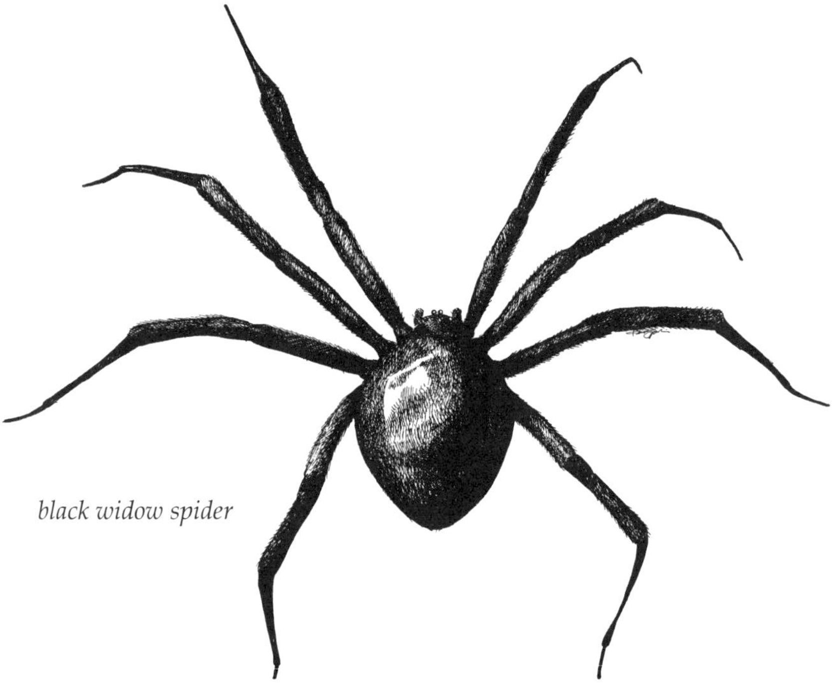

black widow spider

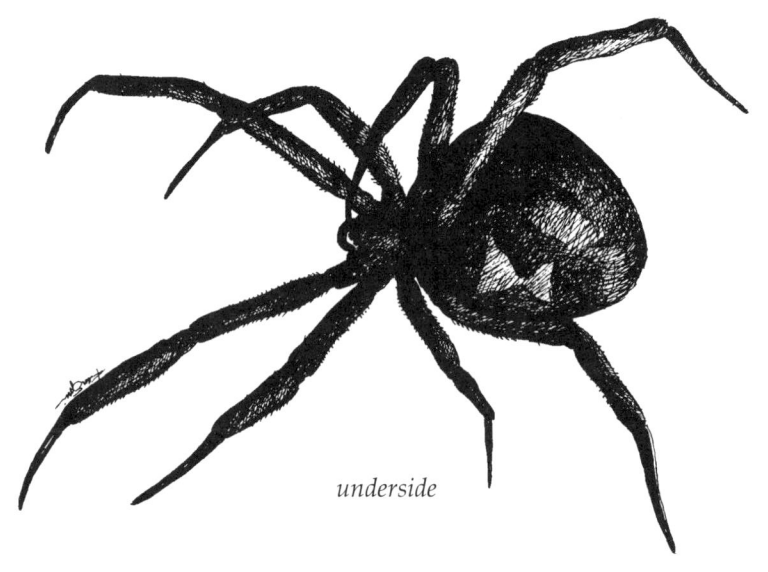

underside

Spider Bites

All spiders have venomous bites, but only two in the Sonoran desert are famous as being dangerous. These are the black widow and the brown recluse. From our experience there are other varieties with devastating bites, which have so painfully added to our list of unpleasant experiences — such as the desert wandering spider.

Black Widow

A black widow bite may or may not produce swelling and pain at the bite site itself. Pain spreads throughout the body, especially in the abdomen and extremities, accompanied by cramping. There may be nausea and vomiting, breathing difficulty, dizziness, ringing in the ears, and sensitivity to noise. Headache, profuse sweating, and alternate dry and wet mouth may occur.

If not treated, in most cases the results of the bite will clear up after a few days of suffering. Small children or adults in a weak state may die. More people die from black widow bites than from rattlesnake bites. The rattlesnakes are generally more terrifying.

Brown Recluse, Cellar, and Desert Wandering Spiders

The true **brown recluse** spider (*Loxosceles reclusa*) does not make a web. It usually spends much of its time under pieces of wood lying loosely on the ground or under boxes in a storage area. I have heard that recluses have six eyes while all other spiders have eight, but I have never looked that close.

The bite of a brown recluse may go unnoticed, because the bite is not painful. However, from the time of the bite the symptoms develop and get worse.

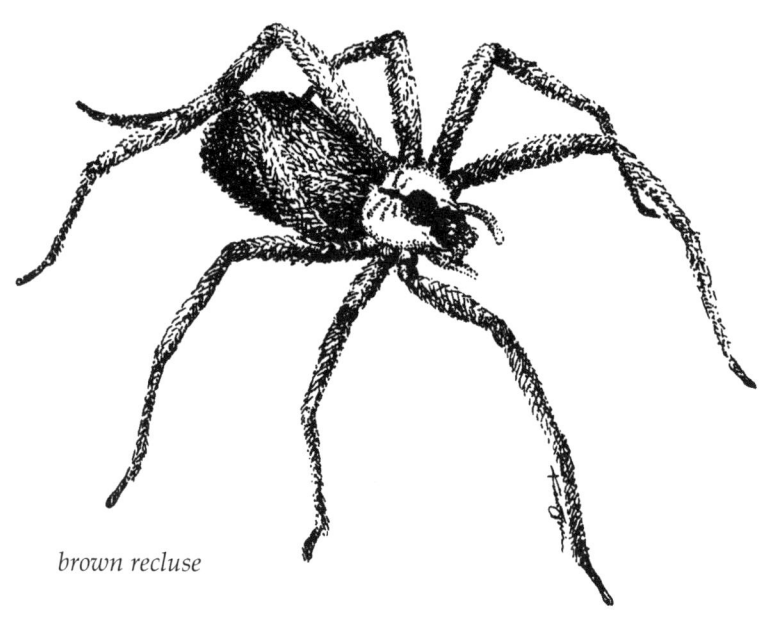

brown recluse

First sign of the bite is likely to be a small red bump that feels hot and itchy and may be painful. The most characteristic symptom of the brown recluse bite is a hard outer ring with a degenerating red, pus-filled center that continues to increase in size, getting wider and deeper. The bite may produce fever, chills, weakness, vomiting, and pains in the joints and muscle tissue. These symptoms will probably occur within 48 hours. If left untreated, the bite may go on increasing in size and suffering for several months.

Currently, the medical treatment is to surgically remove the afflicted area. Fortunately, we have sweeter options for you.

Cellar spiders (family Pholcidae) are often referred to as brown recluses. They have the same "fiddle"-shaped dark silhouette on their back as the true brown recluse, and the same bite with the same results. These spiders have more slender bodies and longer legs, and they make webs. Cellar spiders sometimes live in families of various sizes, adults and babies together.

They prefer to live in the dark corners of a house, under furniture, and in storage rooms. Their bite is similar to that of the true brown recluse.

Cellar spiders are sometimes confused with daddy long legs, which are harmless. Daddy long legs, also called harvestmen (order Opiliones), are arachnids, but they are not spiders.

The **desert wandering spider**, also called the giant crab spider (*Olios fasciculatus*), looks similar to a brown recluse, but it is much larger, and it has furry legs. Desert wanderers do not make webs. I know they are bad news, because I have been bitten by one.

Even though the symptoms may be different with the various types of spider bites, we treat them all in the same way.

Tarantulas & Centipedes

We encounter tarantulas occasionally here at the farm, but I have never received or observed any harm from them. In fact, I have let them crawl up my bare arm on

> Recently, I was bitten three times up under my shirtsleeve by two different western brown recluse (cellar) spiders. Rather than using herbs that I knew would work well, I felt it was a good opportunity to try out some new possible remedies. When one of them worked, I would discontinue it, let the wound fester up again, and then try another.
>
> After nearly a month of this behavior, the poison broke loose and went systemic. I hurt all over so bad I couldn't sleep at night. It felt like this creature in my body had a long-term plan for my demise ... it felt life-threatening at this point.
>
> So, in response to this, I began drinking a tea of Chaparral leaf and Comfrey root. I drank about a gallon and a half in two days, and that completely cured me.

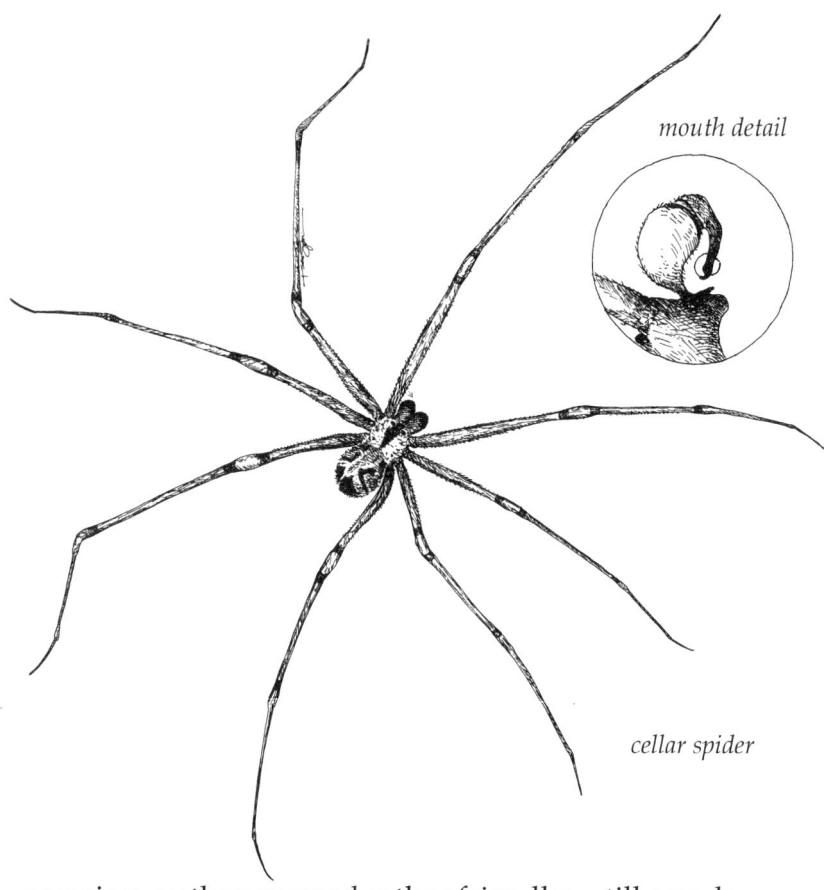

mouth detail

cellar spider

occasion, as they seemed rather friendly ... till one day I noticed the stingers on the fore legs and fangs to bite with. I have heard they can sting, with stingers located at the tips of their fore legs. They can also bite with their impressive-looking fangs. I have read that the sting can be as bad as a wasp sting, or worse for some varieties. If I needed to treat a tarantula sting, I would probably start with our Brown Recluse Remedy and then try other spider bite remedies if that one didn't work.

    Another critter we have never been bit or stung by is the nightmarish desert centipede, which can grow to eight inches long, has powerful pinchers in front, and is reputed to have a stinger in each foot. This may be a myth. If stung, I would probably try treating it like a wasp sting. (See pages 39 through 47.)

Remedies

Poultices & Fomentations

We feel the poultice is the most effective remedy for spider bites and should be applied at any stage—the sooner the better.

When applying poultices over spider bites, cover at least a two-inch diameter area over the bite. Leave on until healed, one to three days. If the healing process seems to slow or stop, then the poultice needs to be changed. Do this as often as needed.

Brown Recluse Remedy: Currently, our favorite poultice for brown recluse and other spider bites is a tincture of three parts Black Walnut bark and one part Chaparral (our Brown Recluse Remedy).

Herb Poultice: For Desert Plantain, Chaparral, or Desert Lavender, use the fresh herb or reconstituted dried herb or powder. For Pasture Bindweed, use a fresh mashed poultice. For Datura, use a stack of the whole leaves placed against the skin. Do not crush the leaves.

> One night while I was sleeping I got bit by a large reddish-brown spider. I woke up with a pain in my wrist and found the spider biting it. I had earlier swatted that spider with a fly swatter and it had gotten away wounded. I suspect it was a desert wanderer. My partner at the time, Angelique, immediately went out to get a Prickly Pear cactus pad. To harvest and prepare the pad took almost 15 minutes. By this time the bite had advanced greatly to a painful, spicy-hot feeling of evil energy moving up my arm at an alarming rate. We taped the pad over the bite. The pain subsided within 15 minutes, and by morning the bite was completely healed. The spider died!

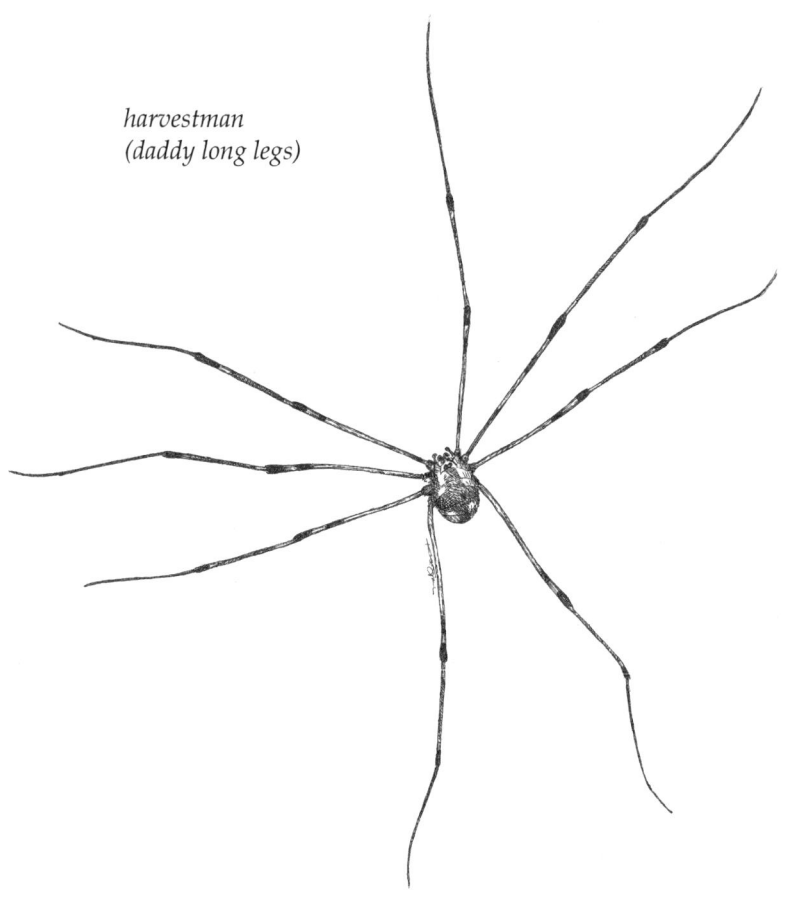

harvestman
(daddy long legs)

Many years ago a friend phoned during the night and said he had been bitten on the hand by a black widow. He had been reaching into an unlit shelf area in the garage to retrieve some auto parts and felt the pain of something biting him. When he pulled his hand out there was a black widow spider still biting him. I recommended that he put on a poultice of Desert Lavender and drink Chaparral tea. The pain went away rather quickly. He experienced a slight upset stomach for a few hours, and then he was back to normal.

Alternatively, tinctures of any of the above plants, except Datura, may be applied with cotton wadding or balls. Tape a handful of the cotton over the bite and then saturate it with the tincture.

Herb Fomentations: Use a cool fomentation of the tea or tincture of Chaparral, Echinacea root, Desert Plantain, or Desert Lavender.

Cactus Poultice: Apply a large Prickly Pear or Hedgehog cactus pad to the bite site. Change as often as needed until the bite is healed.

Bigfoot's Bee/Insect Sting Remedy: Tape a cotton ball or cotton wadding over the bite and apply the tincture to saturate the cotton, until healed.

Black Cohosh Fomentation: Effective but not my first choice.

Herb Teas

If I were in an advanced stage of a venomous spider bite and feeling sick, I would drink one of the following herb teas: Chaparral, Echinacea root, Desert Plantain, Black Cohosh root, or Walnut tree bark.

A man came to me with a brown recluse spider bite that had afflicted an area about 2½ inches in diameter, and asked me if I knew of anything that could help him. He showed me four other places on his body where he had rather large scars where previous bites had been surgically removed.
    We put a poultice of reconstituted Desert Plantain powder over the new bite. The next day it was about 75% healed. We replaced the poultice with another, and did the same again on the third day. After that there was no trace left of the bite.

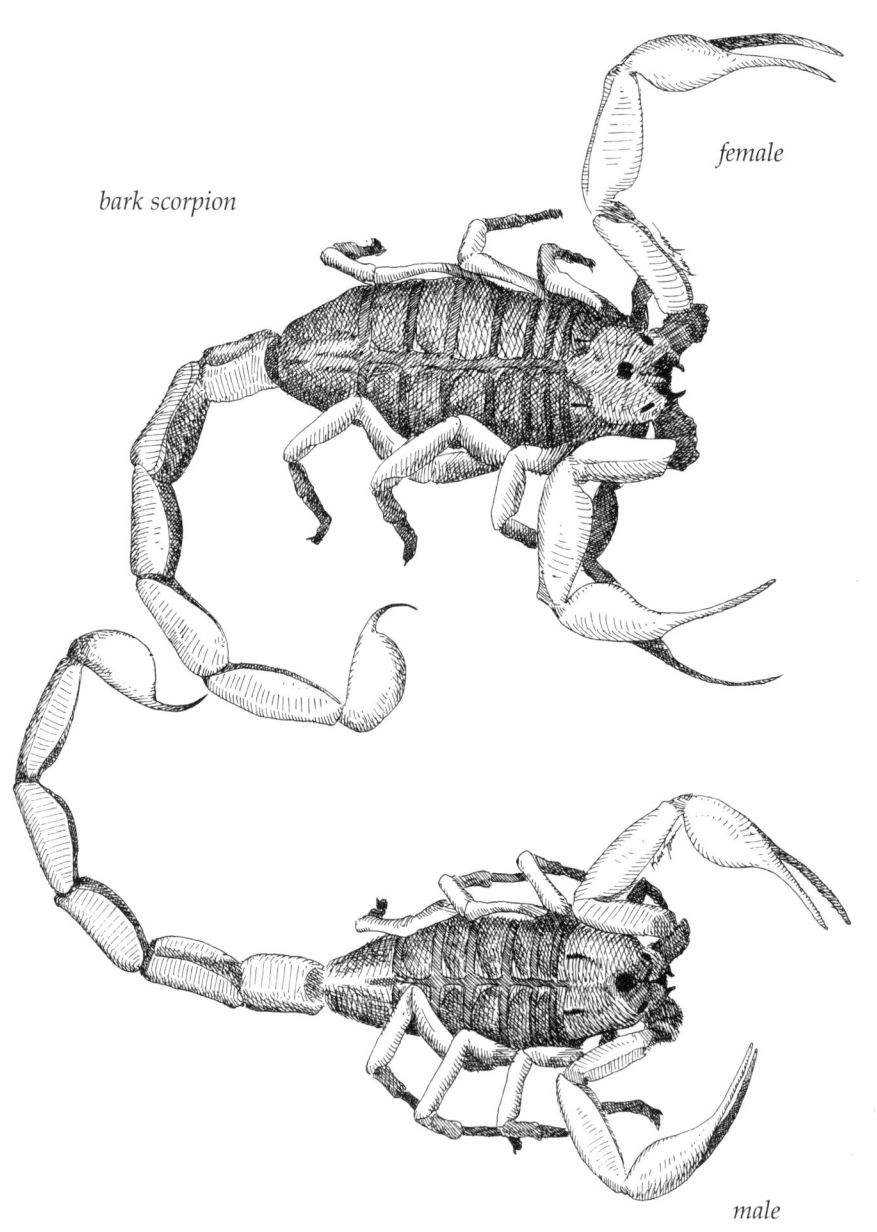

Scorpion Stings

The two basic types of scorpion are the bark scorpion and the rock scorpion. There are several known varieties of each of these. Scorpions sting with the end of their tail; they use their pinchers to hold their prey while they eat.

The **rock scorpion** (see page 26) has thick, sturdy pinchers, and the tail has short, sturdy segments. When resting, it most often holds its tail up over its head. The sting of a rock scorpion is painful. A small amount of localized swelling and redness may occur. The pain, tingling, and numb sensation are most likely to remain localized. The symptoms will last from several hours to a couple of days, taper off to just the numb sensation, and then be gone.

The **bark scorpion** is much more dangerous. One member of the bark scorpion family is the *Centuroides*

Several years ago, during the night, a woman got stung by a bark scorpion in her armpit. It hurt for a short time and then the pain subsided, with numbness and twitching under the skin. She didn't treat it and tried to go back to sleep. Three hours later she was becoming paralyzed and couldn't speak. Her partner woke me up about 3:00 a.m. for assistance.

The woman was making sounds, but we couldn't understand what she was trying to say. She obviously had intense pain throughout her upper body, her chest was constricted, and her heart and lungs seemed to be in trouble. I prepared a Prickly Pear cactus pad and placed it over the sting site. We saw almost instant improvement. She was still suffering but much less than before.

We gave her an oriental acupressure treatment for the lymphatic system, and changed the cactus pad. About 12 hours later she was feeling better.

sculpturatus. This is the deadly variety found in southern Arizona and northern Mexico, including here at our farm. Bark scorpions have thin, frail-looking pinchers and long, thin tail segments compared to the rock scorpion. When resting, bark scorpions lay their tails over to one side.

The young bark scorpion is orange in color. As it grows larger it becomes more a straw color and less orange.

Having received 31 bark scorpion stings, I have noted that they have several different effects. The variety of symptoms includes intense pain at the sting site, similar to that of a continuous burn. The sting hurts like hell for the first hour, subsides for about three hours, and then begins to get worse and worse and worse! As the venom circulates through the body, the pain at the

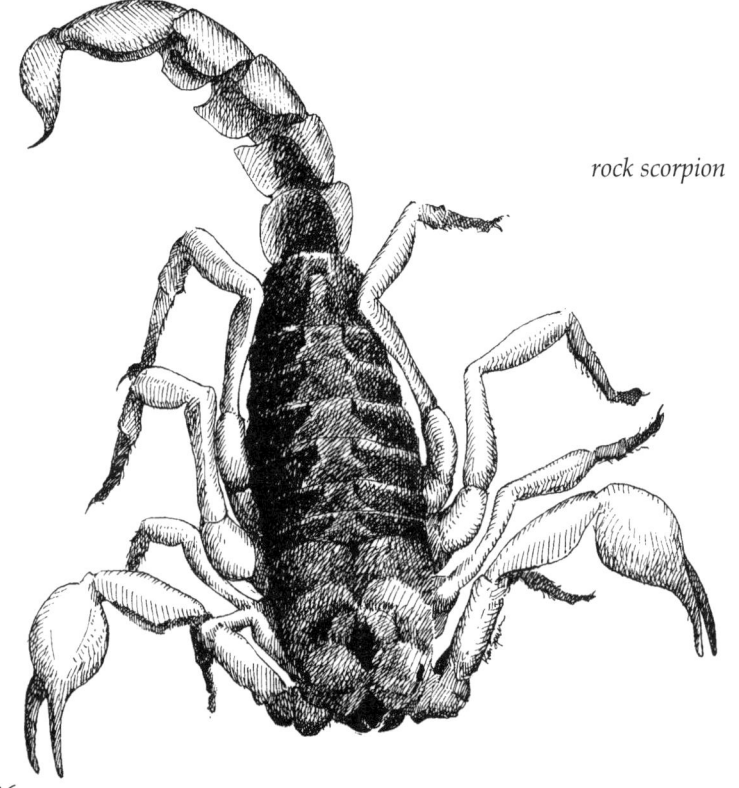

rock scorpion

One evening, while lifting a bale of hay, I was stung by a large bark scorpion on the end of my middle finger. Immediately there was intense prickling pain in the finger. Following a suggestion I had received as an old Indian remedy, I applied the juice from the next to last segment of the scorpion's tail to the sting site as an experiment — although my intuition was shouting at me that this was *not* a good idea! It seemed to help relieve the pain, for a short time, but then the pain got worse.

The sting had occurred at 6 p.m. Around 6:15, I drank a pint of Black Cohosh tea. At 7:00 I soaked the finger in a bowl of Cottonwood leaf mush. By 8:00 the pain in the finger was slight; however, I had an intense headache behind the eyes and in the back of my head. I also had pain and discomfort behind the knees and in the sacrum and elbows.

At 9:00 p.m. I found it necessary to lay down. Yet my body kept moving around, trying to find a comfortable position, but there was none. So, much of the night I sat up. I was too disabled to stand. Sound was irritating, and light hurt my eyes. I also experienced periods of feeling cold. I suffered through the night with restless agitation and pain throughout my body.

About 3:30 a.m. I drank Cottonwood tree bark tea, which seemed to help relieve the headache. After this I found that walking felt good. Then I slept for a while. At around 6 or 7 a.m. a feeling of tightness in my chest and heart seemed to be on the increase. The heart and lung functions seemed threatened. I changed from soaking the finger in Cottonwood leaf mush to Prickly Pear mush. That afternoon, I began feeling free of it. No more scorpion tail juice for me!

While I was drying myself with a towel, a rock scorpion, which had been sleeping in the towel, stung my abdomen. It hurt with burning pain. We applied Prickly Pear cactus pad to the sting area. The pain subsided in a half hour, and then it was gone. Bark scorpions are not that easy.

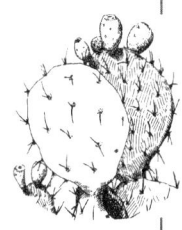

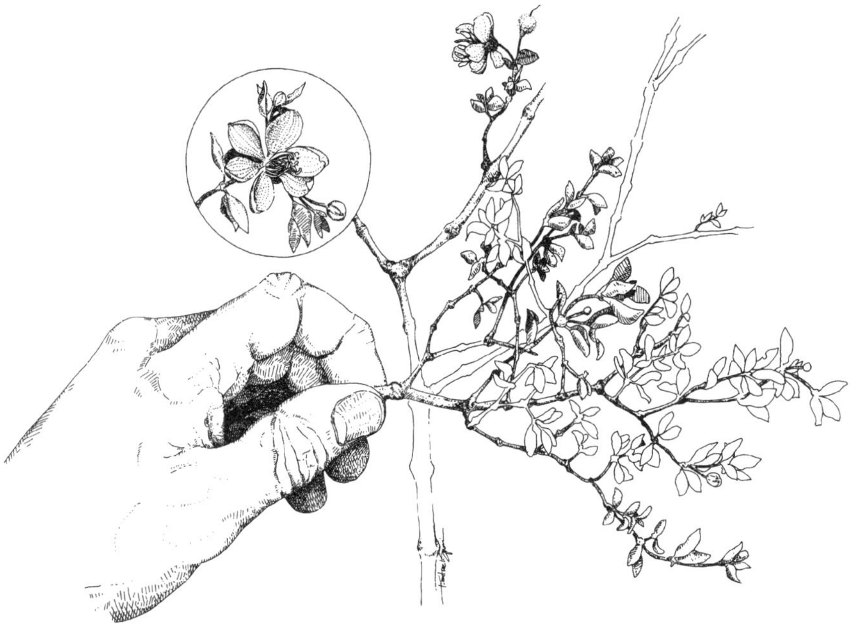

Chaparral

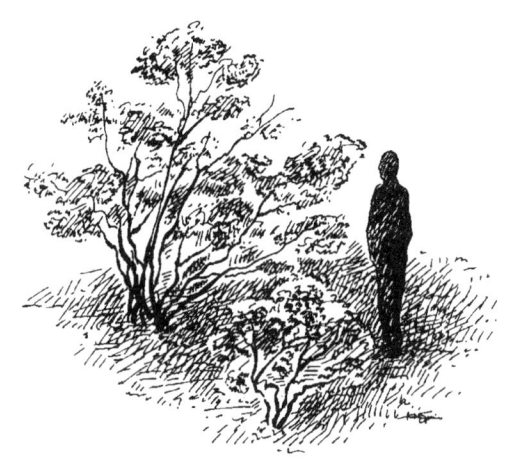

sting site radiates through the body. The pain then is replaced by numbness and tingling. The person may feel nervous twitching, like a scorpion is running up and down under the skin.

Two to six hours after the sting, the person may become sick to their stomach and experience partial paralysis, blindness, convulsions, fever, slurred speech, restriction of the heart, increased heart rate, difficulty breathing, a constricted feeling in the chest, intense headache, and restless agitation. Too sick to stand, the person may try to lay down, but there is no comfortable position. The acute symptoms usually subside within 12 to 48 hours without treatment, but the numbness and tingling may last for weeks.

From experience and observation we know that stings in the fingers and toes are most painful and seem to affect the entire body in a life-threatening way. The areas of the body with thick skin and the fleshy outside areas of the body (like the outside of the thighs and arms and the back) are the least serious areas. The twitching

> Once I was picking up a piece of canvas off the ground when I got stung in the finger. There was intense prickly pain. I ran to the house, poured a tincture of fresh Western Mugwort into a cup, submerged my finger in it, and kept it there. Within 15 minutes it had relieved 80% of the pain, tingling, prickling, and numbness. I was thrilled! I also drank some of the tincture in a cup of water.
>
> I noticed that if I took my finger out of the tincture, the prickling pain returned. Six hours later, I saturated a large piece of cotton wadding and wrapped it around the sting area so I could lay down without spilling the tincture. By morning the finger was normal. All the pain and suffering was kept local in the finger and did not travel to other parts of the body, as it had with other stings. Success!

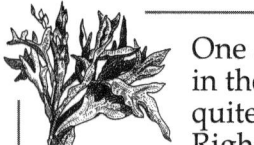

One afternoon Chuckie Chicken got stung in the face by a scorpion. He was still quite young, weighing less than a pound. Right away we gave him diluted tincture of Western Mugwort internally, and then we soaked him in a warm bath of Mugwort tea. By morning he was walking, although somewhat wobbly, and one eye was still shut. Without further treatment, the next day Chuckie was fully recovered. If not treated right away, a chicken would usually die from such a sting.

A friend of mine got stung by a bark scorpion on a finger. He had some water left over from cooking Oak tree nuts (acorns) and submerged the finger in it. This water was high in tannic acid from the acorns. He said that it gave him immediate and lasting relief.

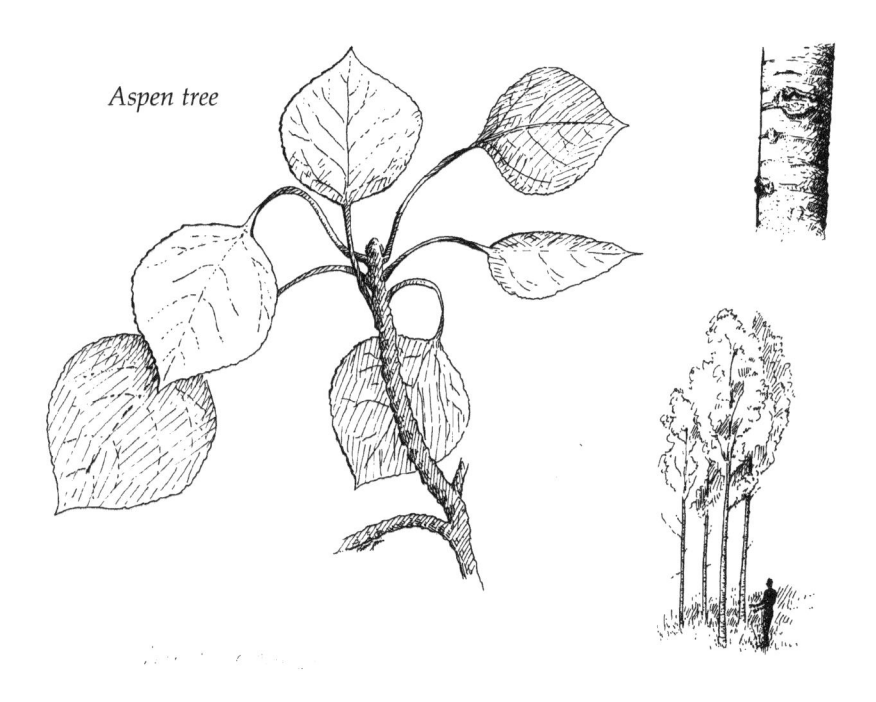

Aspen tree

and numb sensation in these tougher areas is most often experienced without much pain or feeling of threat to the rest of the body. The thin-skinned areas, like under the arms and the armpits, hands, fingers, wrists, feet, toes, neck, and groin, are serious areas. Multiple stings increase the suffering. The bark scorpion is no joke! They can put a person through much suffering and even cause death for children or weak adults.

One characteristic of all bark scorpion stings is that there is little or no swelling at the sting site. For this reason it is important to make a mental note or mark the site of the sting immediately after the occurrence, so that you know where to place your poultice.

Both types of scorpion stings are treated in the same way.

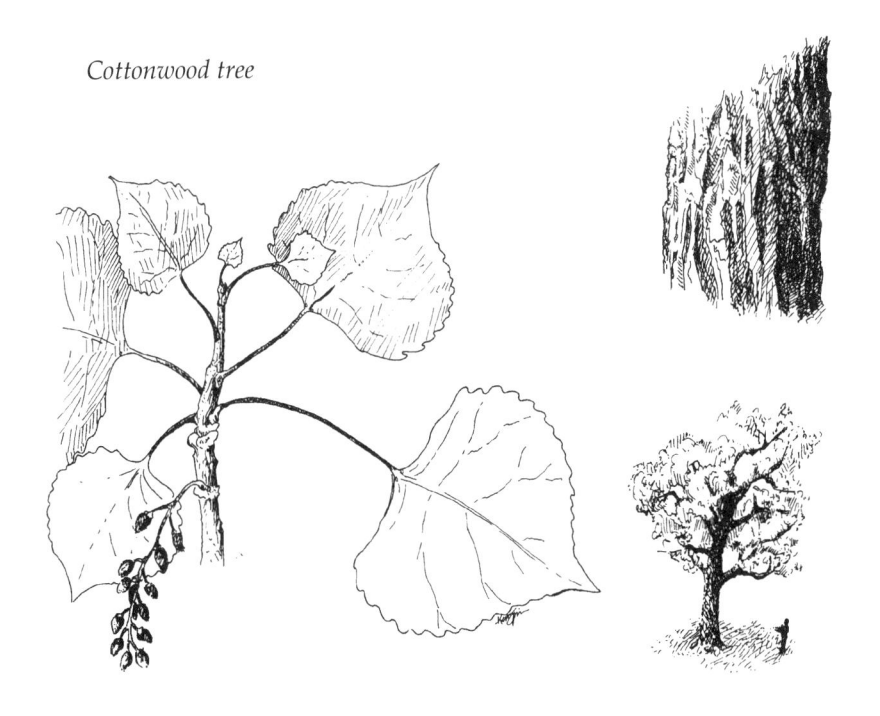

Cottonwood tree

mature plant

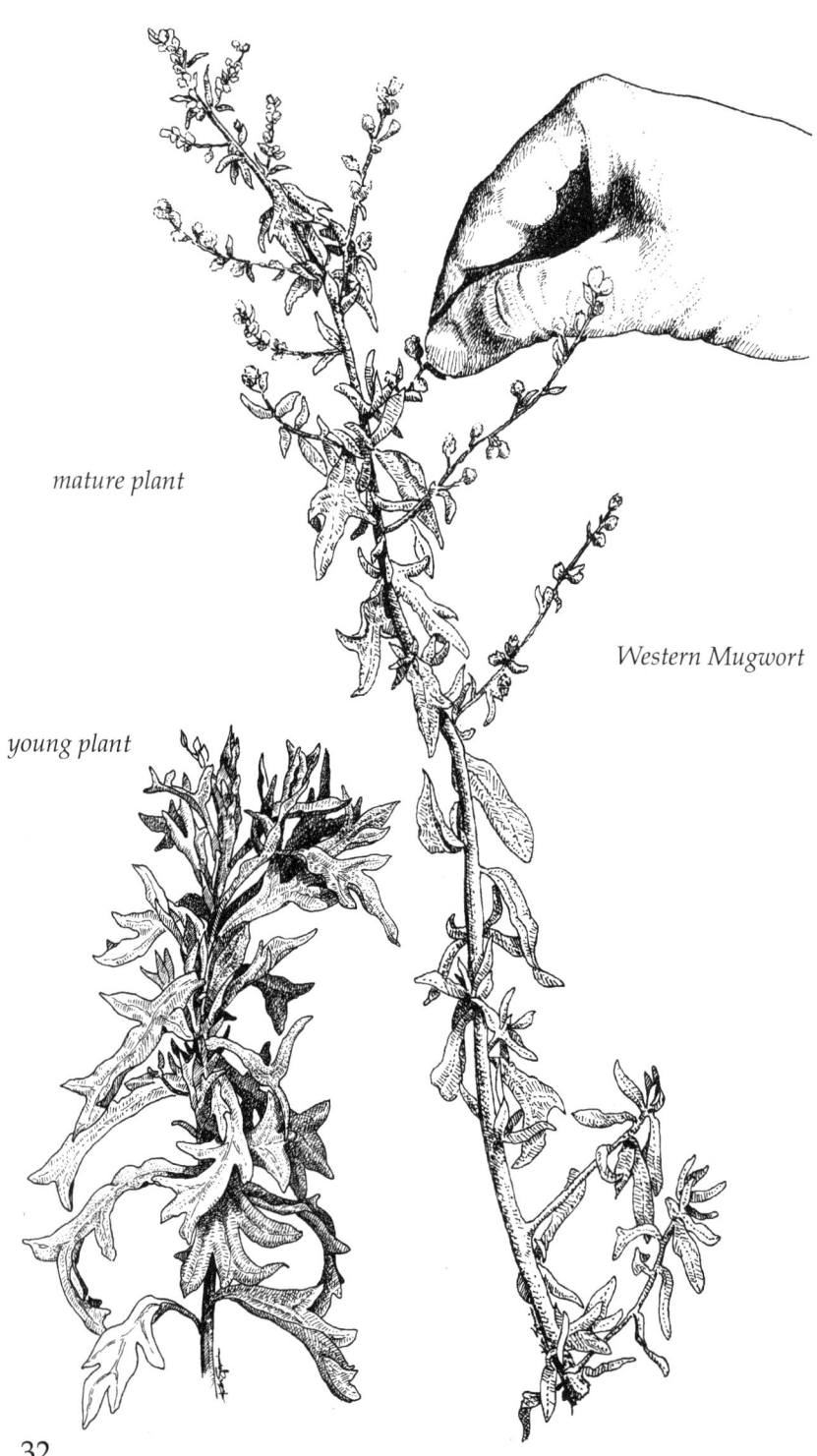

young plant

Western Mugwort

Remedies

It has been a real challenge for me to find a remedy for these #*#*! stings. The treatment that I'm really excited about lately is to submerge my stung finger in a small cup of tincture of fresh Western Mugwort.

Poultices & Fomentations

Western Mugwort Tincture: Soak the afflicted area in tincture of fresh Western Mugwort, or tape a handful of cotton wadding over the sting (to cover approximately a two-inch diameter area), and then saturate it with tincture.

Prickly Pear Cactus: Apply a poultice of Prickly Pear cactus pad. For a sting on a finger or toe, scrape the pulp out of the pad with a spoon and mash or blend it. Soak the whole foot or hand in a bowl of the mashed pulp.

Purslane: Being a common garden plant, Purslane is often a convenient remedy. Mash or chew up a handful of the leaves and stems and apply to the sting. Our friend Mary used this remedy to good effect when a young child in her care was stung.

Cottonwood or Aspen Tree Leaves: Use a large fist-size poultice of the fresh green leaves. For fingers or toes, make a slurry, put in a bowl, and submerge the area.

> While sleeping in bed I was stung by a large bark scorpion on the outside of my lower leg. It hurt for a moment and then began to twitch as though a scorpion was running up and down underneath my skin. There was also a feeling of numbness. I put a large poultice of bruised Cottonwood tree leaves over the sting site and went back to sleep with no further event. If the sting had been on my foot or a finger, I believe it would have been much worse.

Castor plant

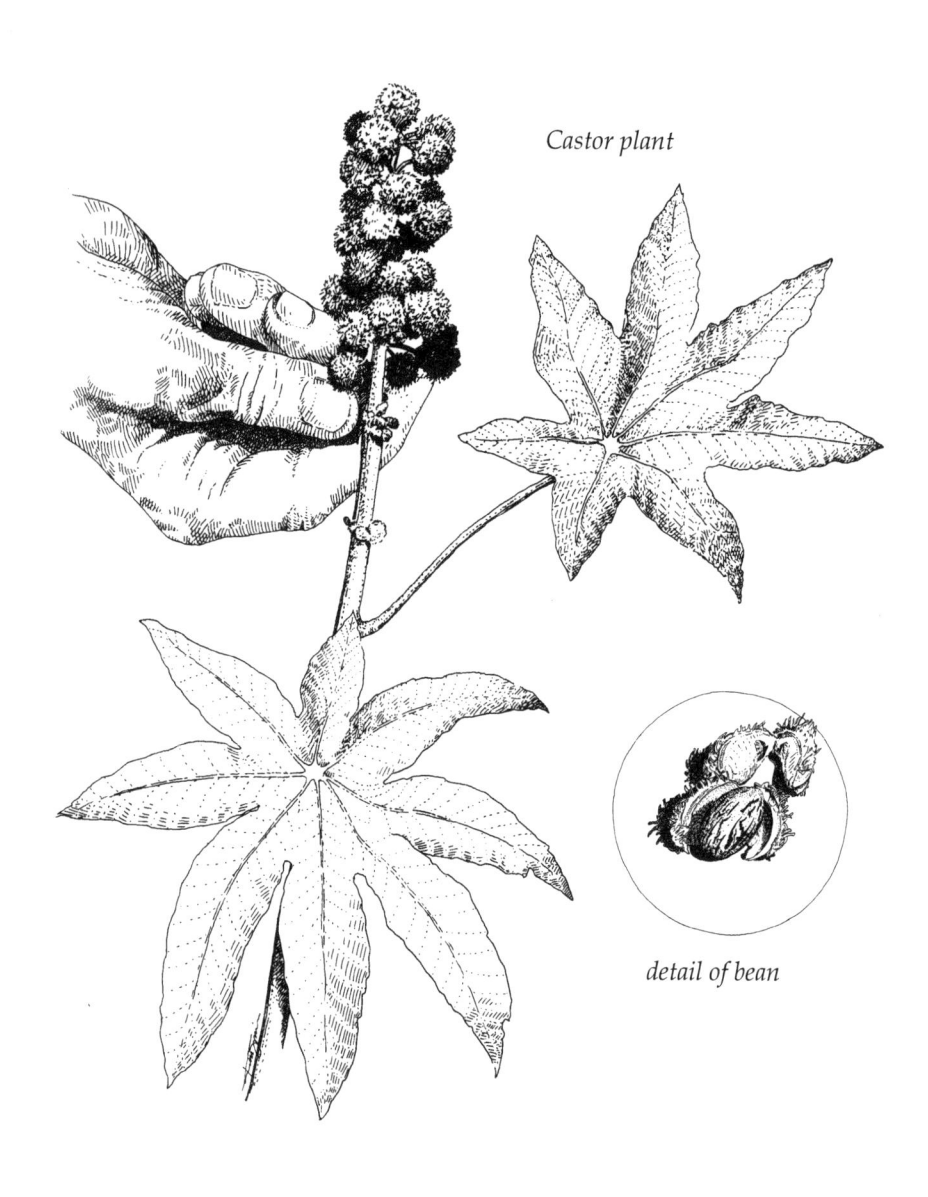

detail of bean

I recently got stung in the groin area by a bark scorpion. This is a vulnerable and potentially dangerous area to be stung.
    I applied a rag saturated with Castor bean oil and kept it on for about six hours, with excellent results. The wound felt comforted by this poultice, and the pain subsided. This is a good remedy.

Castor Oil: Cover the sting site with a cotton bandage that has been saturated with Castor oil. This remedy has worked quite well for me.

Chaparral and Clay: Steep a good handful of dry Chaparral herb in a pint of hot water, to make a super strong tea. Use that tea to moisten dry clay or dirt. Allow it to cool. Pack it on over the sting as a poultice. This sounds good, though I haven't tried it yet. If you don't have clay or dirt, use a cotton cloth.

Herb Teas

Use Western Mugwort (best), Desert Plantain, Chaparral, or Black Cohosh. Drink one cup immediately and then one cup every two to three hours, as needed.

Lemon

A Mexican man once told me that his remedy for scorpion stings was to drink the diluted juice of twelve lemons. Probably not all at once.

Urine

Urine is the most popular remedy used in India for snake bites. It is believed that a person's urine becomes a homeopathic remedy after venom enters the blood. It might work for scorpion stings, too. See page 77.

Indian Lore

I was told, first cut off the stinger segment of the scorpion. Now cut off the next segment and squeeze the juice of it onto the sting. I tried this once and only once. Much suffering resulted. *Not recommended! Don't do it!*

female

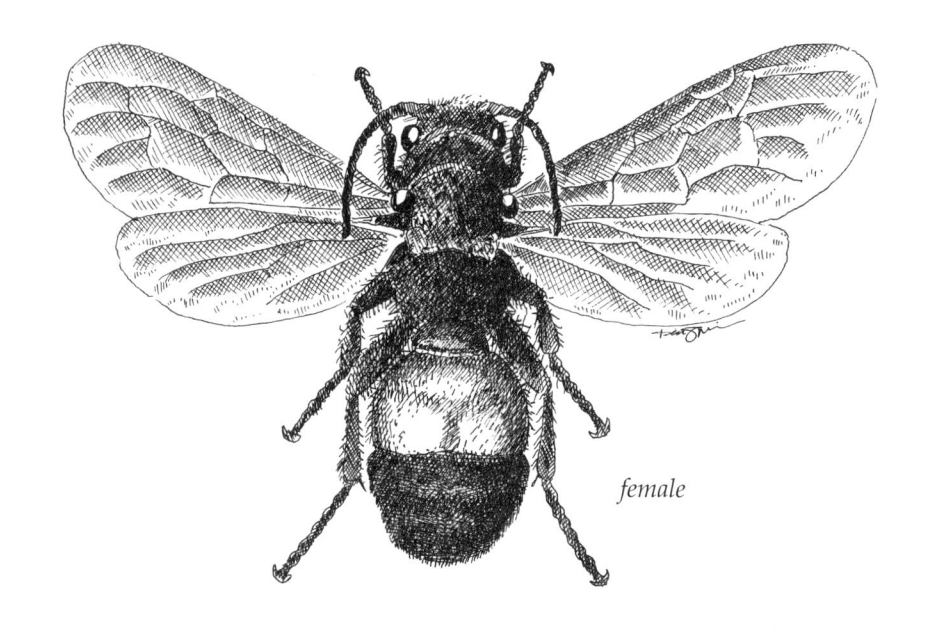

velvet ant

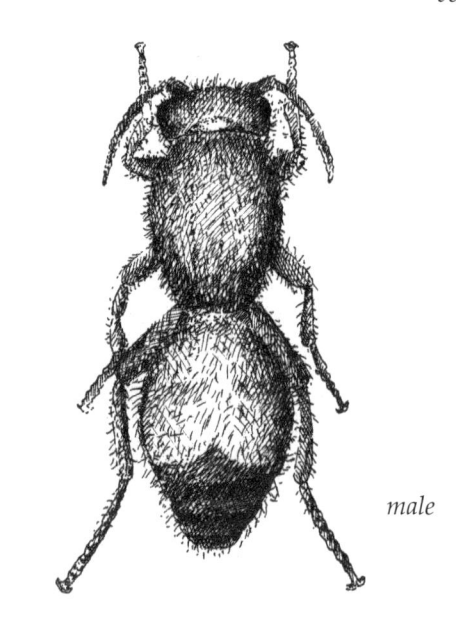

male

Bee, Ant, and Wasp Stings

Bees, ants, and wasps most often sting in defense of their homes (hives) or when trapped in our hair or clothing. They inflict a startling pain. Get away quickly.

Instant pain draws instant attention to the situation. The first symptom after the pain is usually a white swelling with a red dot in the center. Later the swelling turns red and the pain subsides; however, do not ignore the need for treatment at this point. The swelling may increase the following day, accompanied by increased itching. This may continue and get a lot worse for several days if not treated. Do not rub or scratch, as this would compound the swelling and spread the poison.

Ants are wingless wasps and pinch only to hold on while they drive in their stinger and venom. With ants, it is not so much the bite but the sting that hurts. Most Southwest desert ants deliver a severe sting that should be treated like a bee sting.

People who are allergic to insect stings may experience an extreme reaction (anaphylactic shock), characterized by breathing difficulty, an itchy sensation in the throat and/or lungs, an inflamed and itchy sensation around the neck, swollen eyelids, profuse watery mucus running out of the nose, and possible loss of consciousness, which may lead to death of the body.

Desert Tobacco

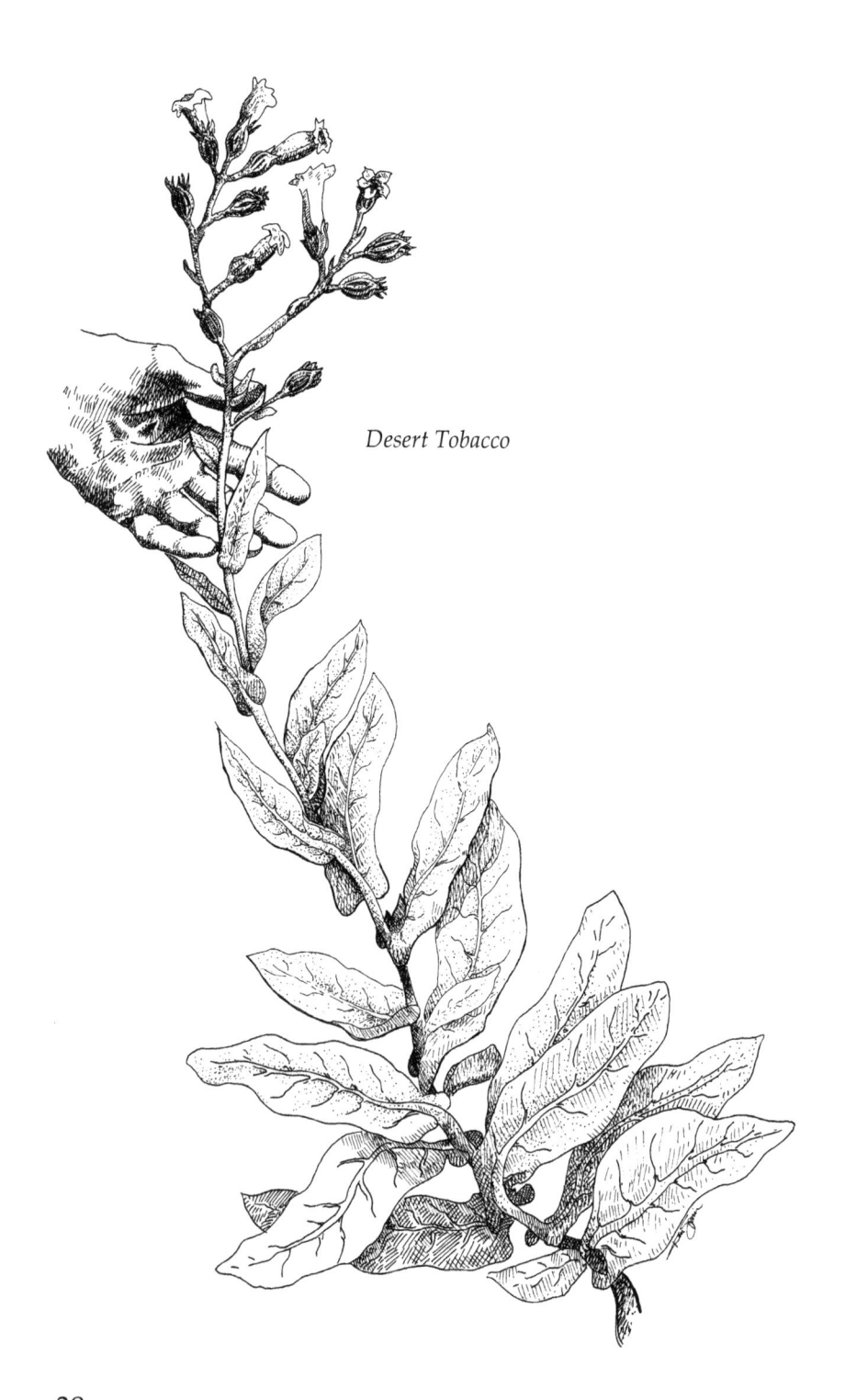

Remedies

First, remove the stinger. Honeybees are the only insects likely to leave their stinger behind. If there is a stinger in the wound, do not try to remove it by pinching with your fingers to pull it out. There is a venom sack on the end of the stinger, and if you pinch it you will inject all of the venom into the body. It is better to flick it out with the blade of a knife or grab the stinger with tweezers below the venom sack. The venom sack is a little grayish-white sack about the size of a poppyseed, with the stinger embedded in the skin. The longer the stinger is left in the skin the more venom is injected into the body, so it is important to remove it quickly.

All of these stings get treated about the same. For a mild case, a poultice is all you need.

Poultices & Fomentations

Bigfoot's Bee/Insect Sting Remedy: First tape a piece of cotton over the area (a one-inch cotton ball or a piece of wadding about that size), and then saturate the cotton with the remedy.

> Once, a bear broke into our bee hives and smashed them up real bad. As I attempted to repair the damage, the bees fiercely attacked me and stung right through my protective clothing. I discovered the meaning of the phrase "loaded for bear"! I was stung so many times that it seemed futile to apply poultices to each sting. My body really hurt! I drank a pint of Black Cohosh tea. A half hour later I was feeling much better, and three hours later I was done with it; no further problem. That was quite an achievement for me because I'm usually allergic to these stings.

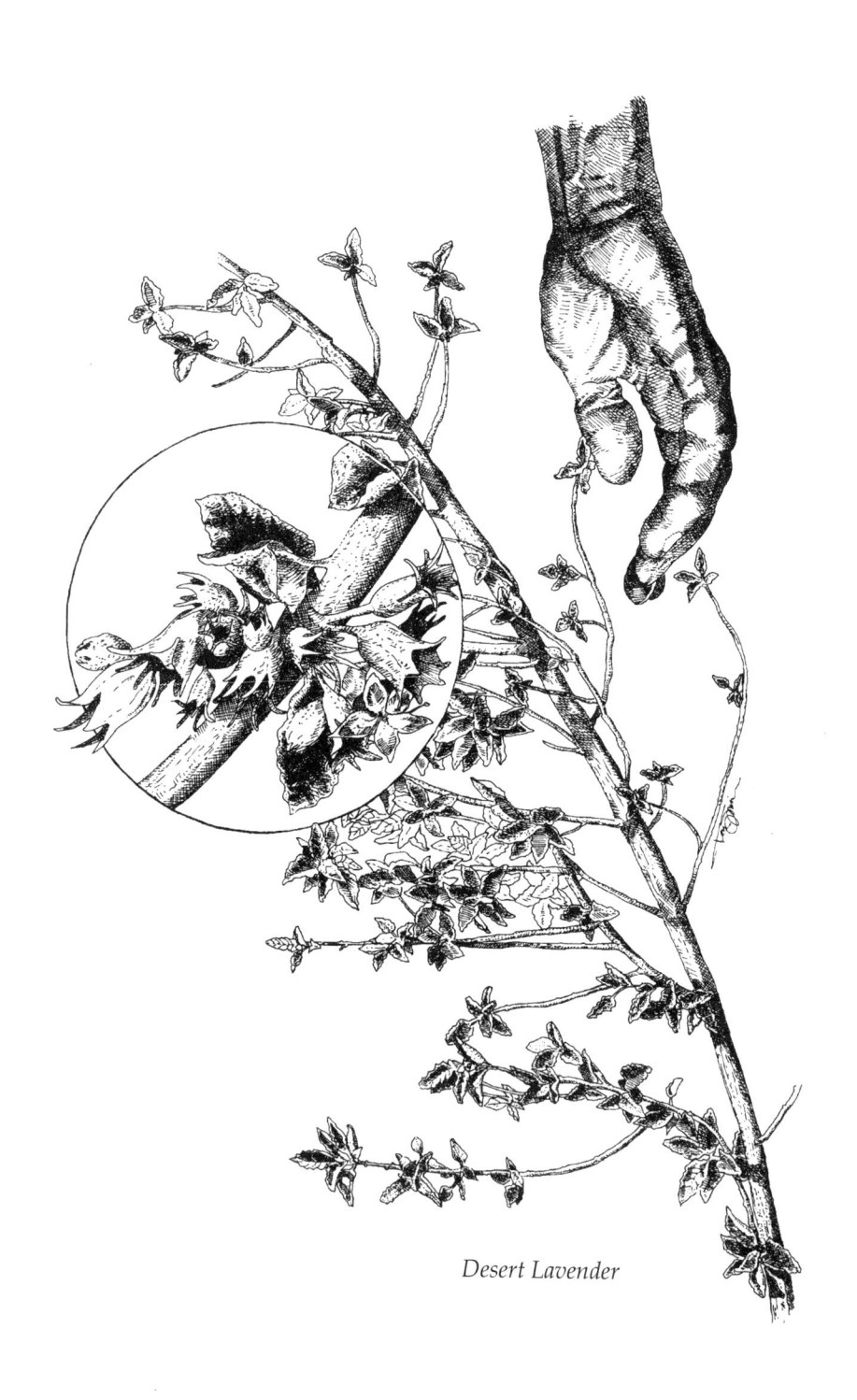

Desert Lavender

Desert Tobacco or Tree Tobacco (a closely related plant)**:** For external use only, a fresh leaf crushed and taped over the sting is marvelous.

Desert Lavender: Apply before the white bump turns red. This only takes five to ten minutes, maximum. The poultice should have a moist, doughy consistency and should be taped onto the wound. The best way is to chew the fresh, dried, or powdered leaf. This may be an unpleasant experience because of the taste, but the small amount that is swallowed seems to help fight the venom.

Prickly Pear or Hedgehog Cactus: Refer to page 69 for instructions to make a poultice from a Prickly Pear cactus pad and page 71 for a Hedgehog cactus.

Sand Spurge: The fresh milky juice of Sand Spurge may be helpful. You will find that when you break off a little stem, a drop of milky sap appears. Place this drop on the sting. Repeat the process until it is well covered. Sand Spurge is related to papaya, which also works.

During an outdoor plant identification class in the desert near Tucson, one of the students got stung by a big red desert ant. Rather quickly the lymph glands in the groin began to swell. Not remembering that we had just studied a plant that could help, I ran off to the truck to retrieve some Desert Lavender I kept in it. In the ten minutes I was away on the rescue mission, one of the students gathered some Four Wing Salt Bush seeds, chewed them until moist, and applied them to the sting. By the time I returned the swelling had subsided.

Purslane

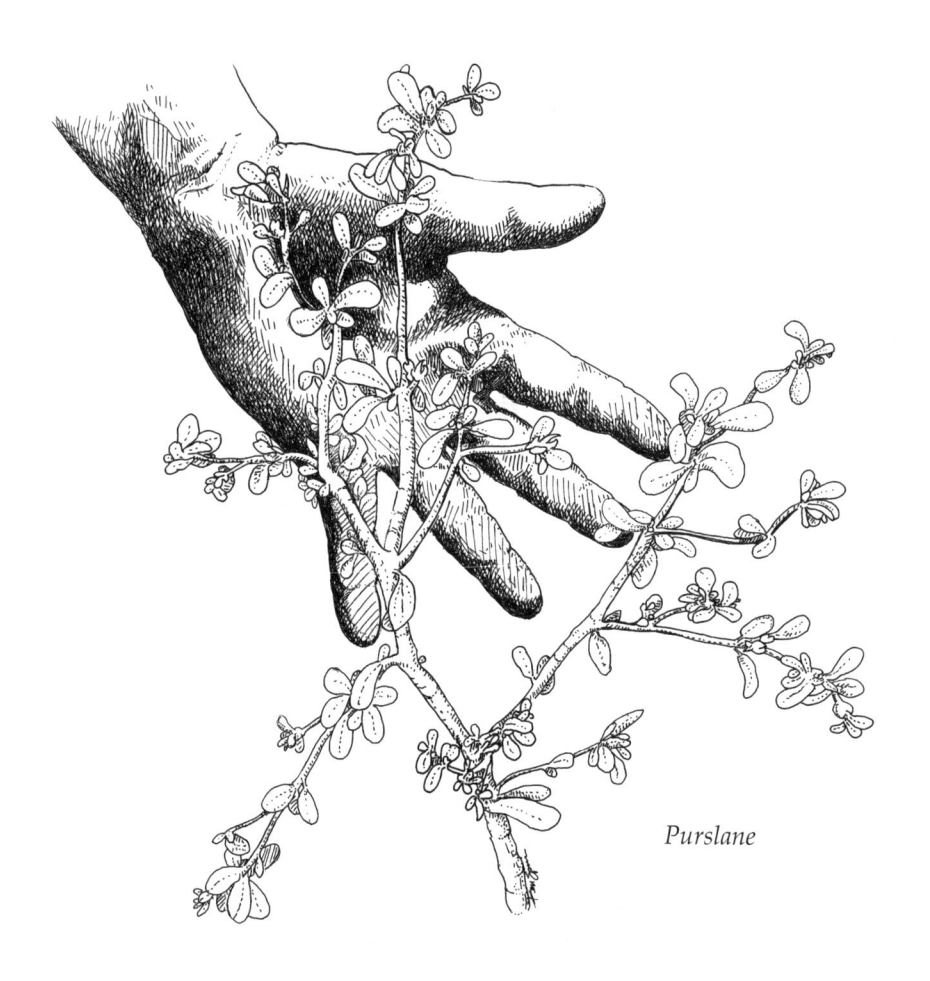

Purslane: This plant is a soft, juicy, rounded, prostrate-growing edible garden weed. I first discovered this use of it when, while weeding my garden, I grabbed a tarantula wasp hidden in the weeds. Wow! It really hurt! Knowing how cool and juicy Purslane is, I quickly chewed some and applied it to the sting. The pain subsided almost instantly.

Turpentine Brush Tincture: This is currently our favorite remedy for swollen and itchy ant stings, especially those of the little brown wood-eating ants that smell like turpentine or pineapples when crushed. Their sting is not painful at first, but it gets worse and the swelling can continue for weeks if untreated.

Other good poultices are fresh or reconstituted Desert Plantain, Four Wing Salt Bush roots or seeds, fresh Cottonwood or Aspen tree leaves, fresh Chickweed, turpentine, mud, or domestic tobacco.

At work as a carpenter, I picked up a board and got stung in the hand by a bee that was on the board. I applied mud, the pain subsided, and I continued working. However, the constant use of my hand aggravated the sting. About two hours later the swelling had increased so much that I had to quit work. Soon the arm was swollen up to the armpit, and I had a sensation of heat, itching, and some pain, accompanied by swollen glands. It looked like I was heading for disaster. I applied an enormous poultice of Desert Plantain (powder of the dried plant reconstituted with water). I kept that on, moist, for about a day and a half, until the symptoms disappeared.

Ephedra

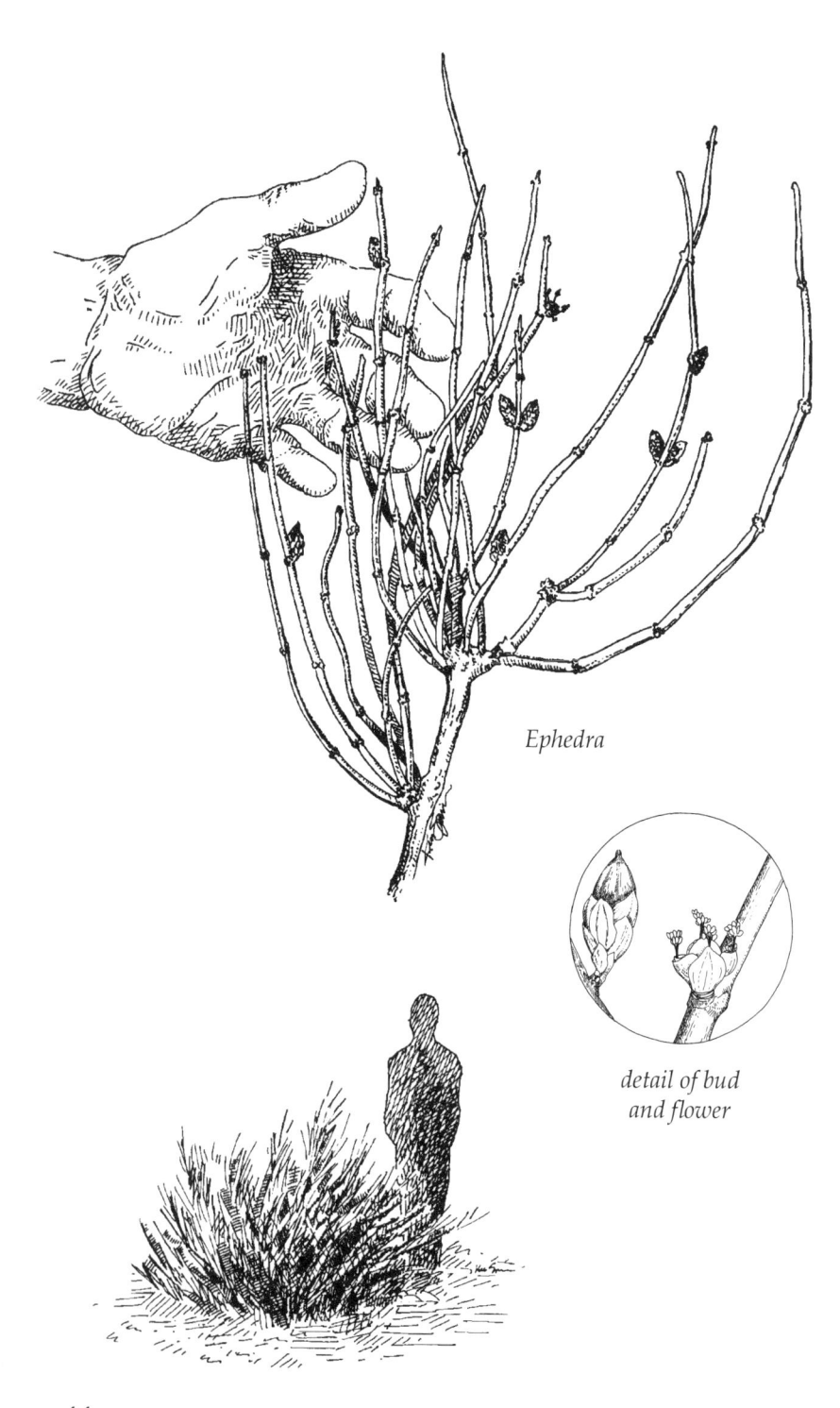

detail of bud and flower

Herb Teas

Use Black Cohosh or Western Mugwort. I would drink at least a cup of this tea and more as needed till I was feeling good again. Desert Plantain, Echinacea, and Chaparral are also good teas for insect bites.

Urine

Urine is the most popular remedy used in India for snake bites. It is believed that a person's urine becomes a homeopathic remedy after venom enters the blood. This remedy may work for insect stings as well. See page 77. Worth trying if it's all you've got.

> **At our place, we use Bigfoot's Bee/Insect Sting Remedy, which we apply with great success. It is simplest to use.**

> One late summer's day while driving down a country road, I tried to get a honeybee off the inside of the window and outside to freedom. Instead of cooperating, it stung me. I stopped the car, got out, and looked for a remedy. I found myself attracted to Desert Tobacco. I crushed some leaves to express the juice onto the sting and held the crushed leaves there for a few minutes. The sting vanished faster than any I'd experienced thus far.

Chickweed

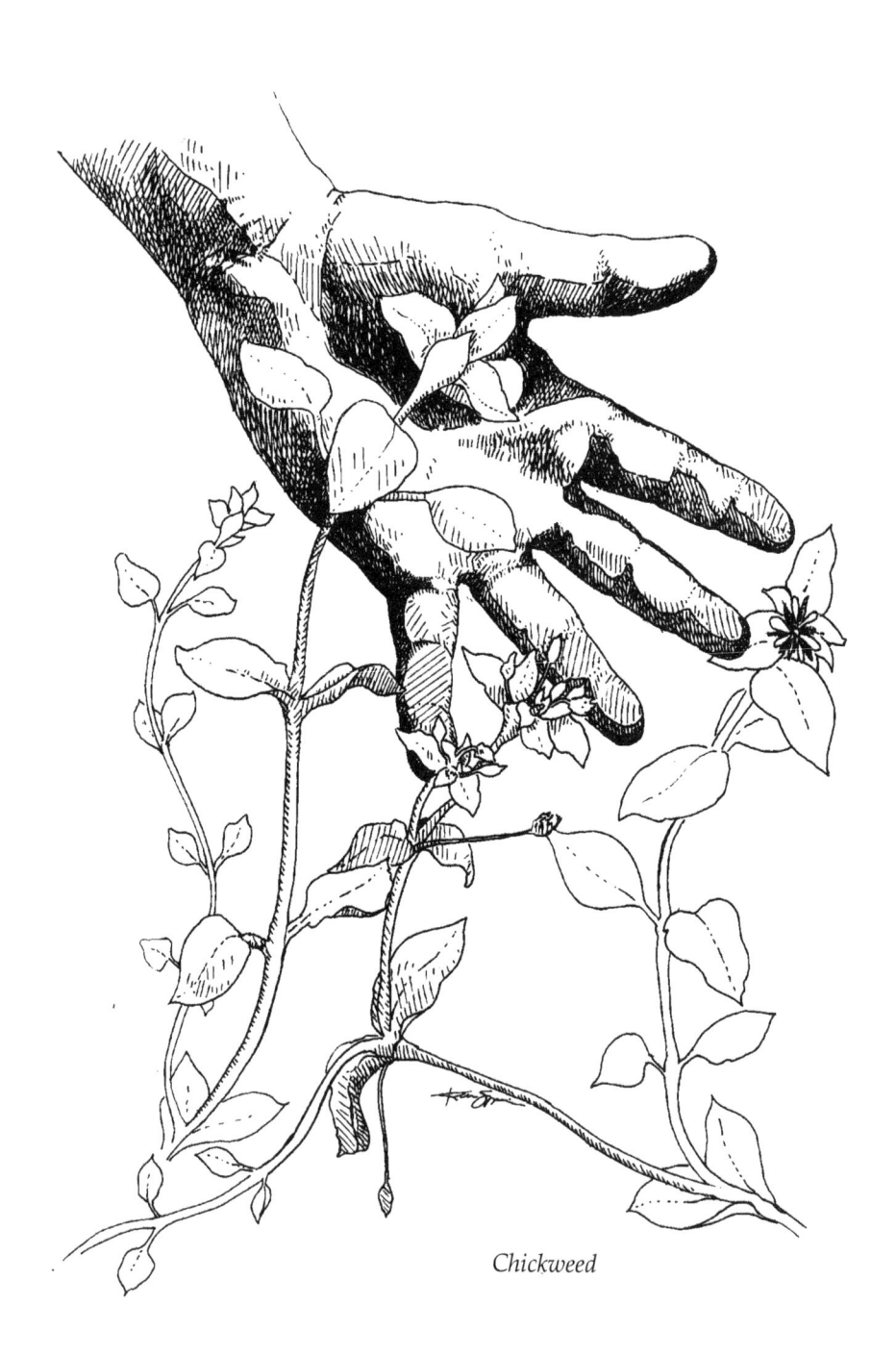

Allergic Reaction (Anaphylactic Shock)

If a severe allergic reaction takes place, I apply one of the recommended poultices. In addition, I would give the person a tea such as Black Cohosh, Western Mugwort, or Echinacea. All of these have worked well for me in the past in this situation and would be my first choice. If these were not available, I would try Valerian, Fennel seed, Catnip, Motherwort, Cottonwood bark, Chamomile, Chaparral, or Ephedra.

I have treated several cases of severe allergic reaction with total success using these remedies.

During a plant study class on Mt. Lemmon, one of the students stepped on a yellow jacket nest. We ran down the mountain and the bees followed us all the way to the parking lot. We all got stung at least twice. It was a great opportunity to try out a variety of remedies. Prickly Pear cactus worked the best of what we had. One of the students went into anaphylactic shock. She drank Black Cohosh tea, which almost immediately reversed the symptoms. All recovered well.

Datura

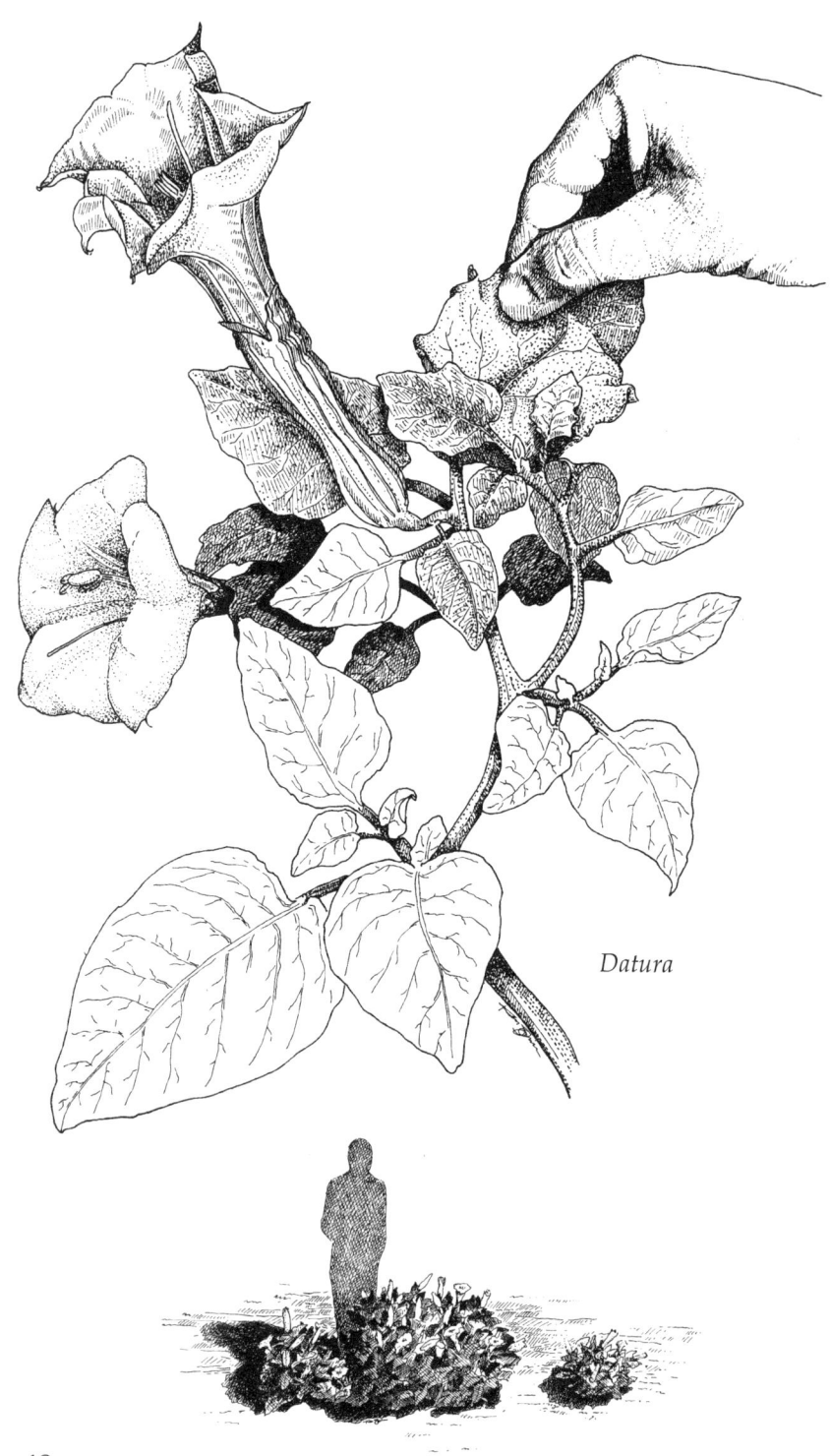

Other Insects

Mosquitoes, Gnats, and Flies

For mosquitoes, gnats, and flies, our favorite remedy is to apply a tincture of one part Chaparral and three parts Black Walnut bark (our Brown Recluse Remedy). We also sometimes use a tincture of Western Mugwort, Desert Plantain, or Camphor weed, or a poultice of fresh Yarrow leaf, Camphor weed, or Desert Plantain. We chew or mash up the leaves and tape them onto the bite. Chewed-up Oak leaf or Western Mugwort also has worked. Usually the simplest thing to do is apply a tincture.

The fresh juice from the stems of the Datura plant works on insect bites, but **do not put the Datura in your mouth!** Datura is poisonous when taken internally, so simply squeeze the juice out of a leaf stem onto the bite. Do this in the morning before the flowers close. Why? Because that's the only way it works.

Scabies

Scabies is a contagious skin infection caused by a super tiny mite that takes up residence and raises families under the surface of the skin. It is very itchy, especially at night. Scabies is distinguished by a straight line, almost like a scratch, with tiny red welts in a row along the line. Scabies spreads rapidly and is easily transferred to others.

The first remedy that we tried that worked was powdered sulfur mixed with Vaseline rubbed onto the afflicted area. My greatest confidence remains with Green Gentian, as for lice (see below).

detail of flower

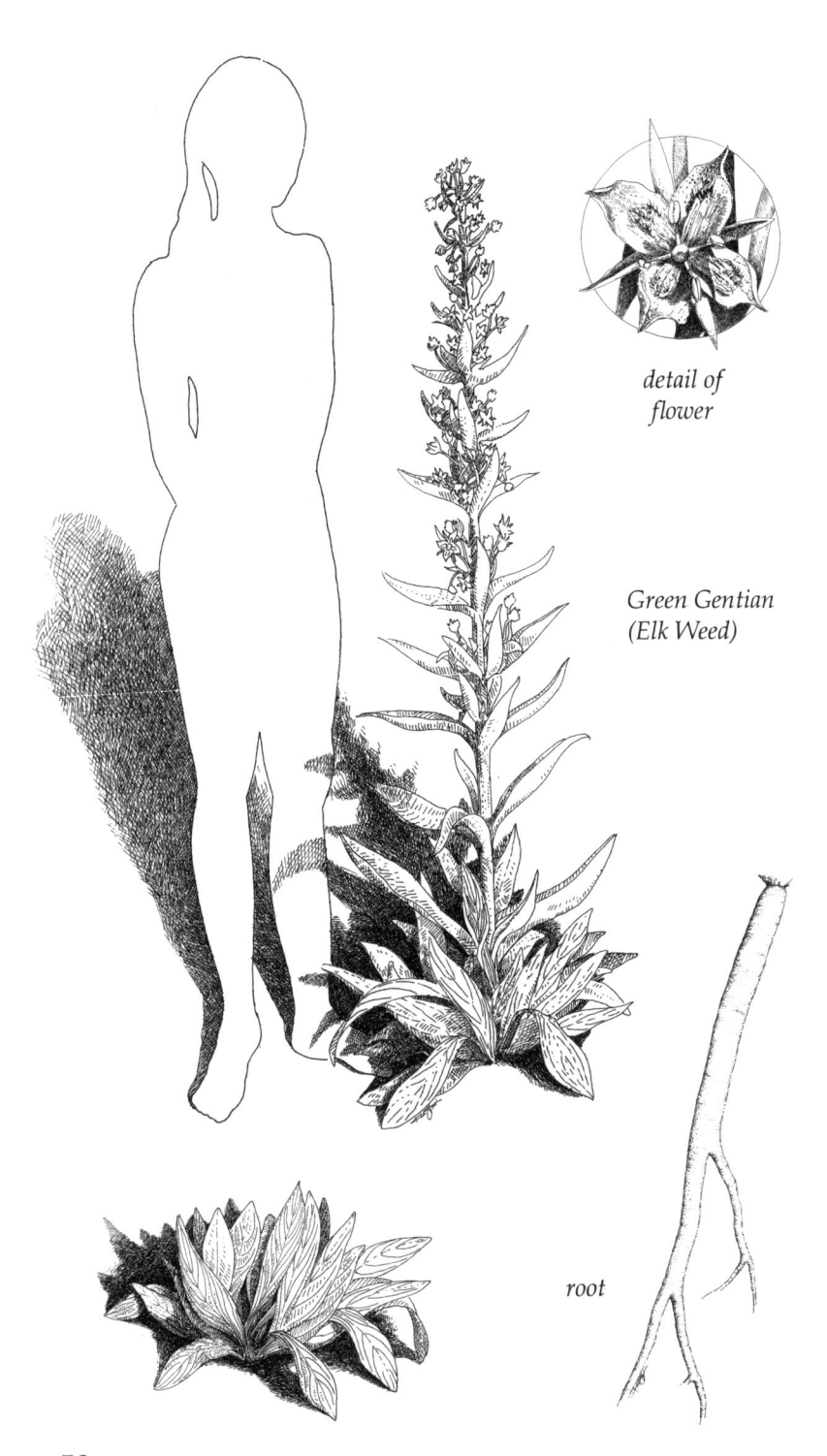

Green Gentian
(Elk Weed)

root

Lice

In the mid 1980s there was an outbreak of head lice all over Arizona. Lice are parasitic bugs that live in the hair and suck blood from the skin. Their eggs are called nits — thus we discovered the meaning of "nit-picking." We made an alcohol tincture of the dried and powdered root of Green Gentian, mixed in some vegetable oil, and rubbed this into our hair and scalp. We left the solution on all day and then washed it out with shampoo and hot water. All the lice were gone, and the nits too. A great success!

Fleas and Ticks

For bites from fleas we use Bigfoot's Bee/Insect Sting Remedy, a Prickly Pear cactus pad poultice, or a tincture of Desert Plantain or Echinacea root. Flea bites can carry some really nasty germs, like plagues and rabies. I suggest that you treat them rather than ignore them. Ticks may carry the dreaded Lyme disease.

If you find a tick buried in your skin, try to get it out. I have always just pulled them out. Some people like to put a lighted match up to their butt, or drown them in rubbing alcohol. After removing the tick, it would be wise to apply some antiseptic. I use a tincture of Desert Willow leaf, Walnut bark, or Chaparral. Plain rubbing

---

One night while out on a camping trip, I picked up a skunk that was terrorizing my friends. Fleas jumped off the skunk and bit me. The bites got immediately infected. There was a deadly plague among the animals that year. I felt like I might have been getting it. I found a Prickly Pear cactus and put a poultice over each bite. The bites were gone by daybreak and I had no further problem.

Desert Willow

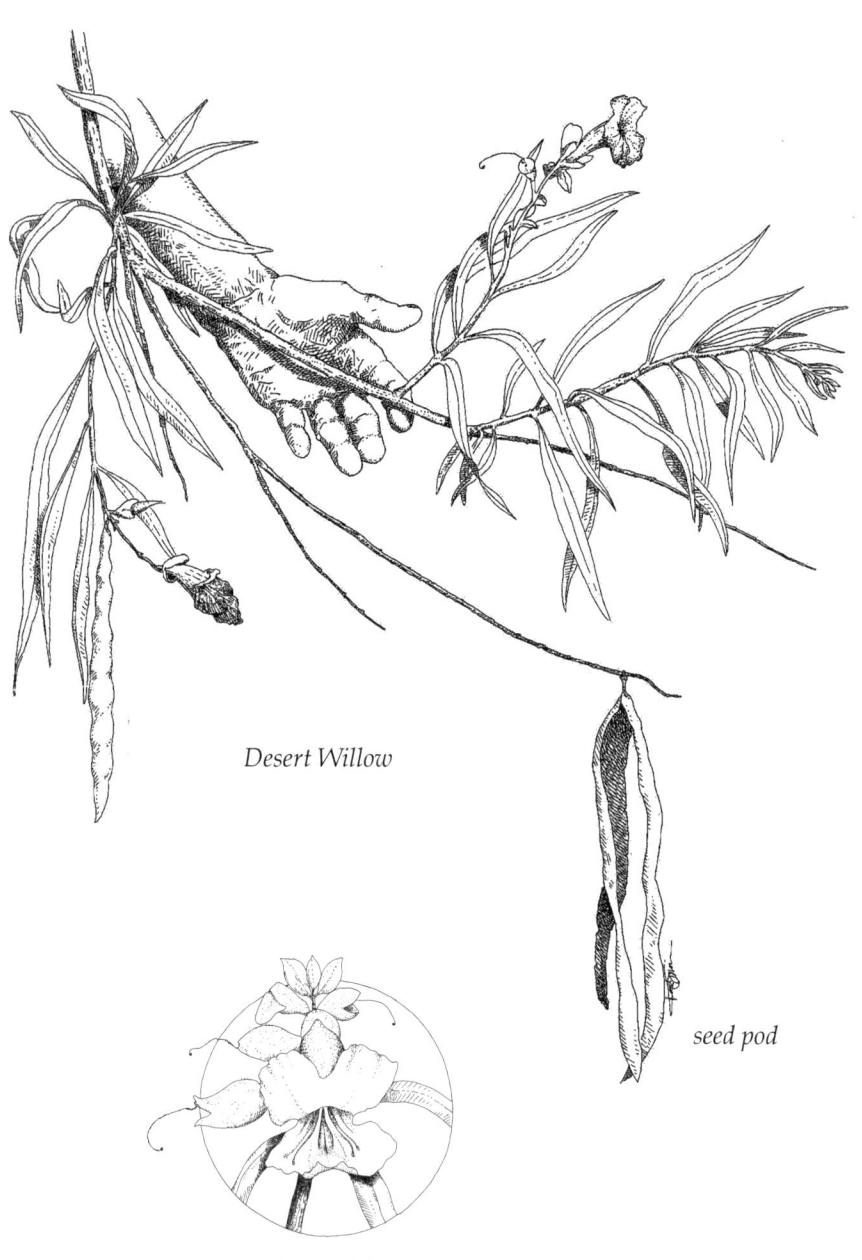

seed pod

detail of flower

alcohol (isopropyl) might do okay. If Lyme disease were to set in, I would go big on Echinacea root, Chaparral, or Desert Willow bark internally.

Chiggers

A Southern curse. These tiny, tiny tick-like insects (the larval stage of a family of mites), red in color, burrow into the skin. We usually contract them by walking through or sitting in moist grass or weeds, especially when the body is hot and sweaty. Actually seeing one in the grass is nearly impossible; they are too tiny.

After exposure to a chigger area, take a cool shower or bath and scrub the skin with soap, as it seems that the minute pests do not burrow in right away, or at least do not get a good hold into their host immediately. An effective preventive measure is to dust your legs with powdered sulfur before going into a chigger zone.

Chiggers usually take up housing in warm, soft areas, such as behind the knees, in the crotch, under the waistband, and under the breasts and arms. The area will swell up and have a stinging, burning, itching feeling. To see the chigger, pinch the swelling until it turns white. The minuscule red dot in the center is the chigger. A magnifying glass would be of great assistance.

To get rid of them, with a small piece of gauze rub tincture of Camphor weed vigorously into the site. Or crush a leaf of Camphor weed or Western Mugwort and tape it over the swelling. Water Pepper applied externally is also very helpful.

We make a good chigger remedy for sale. It is a tincture of Water Pepper and Camphor.

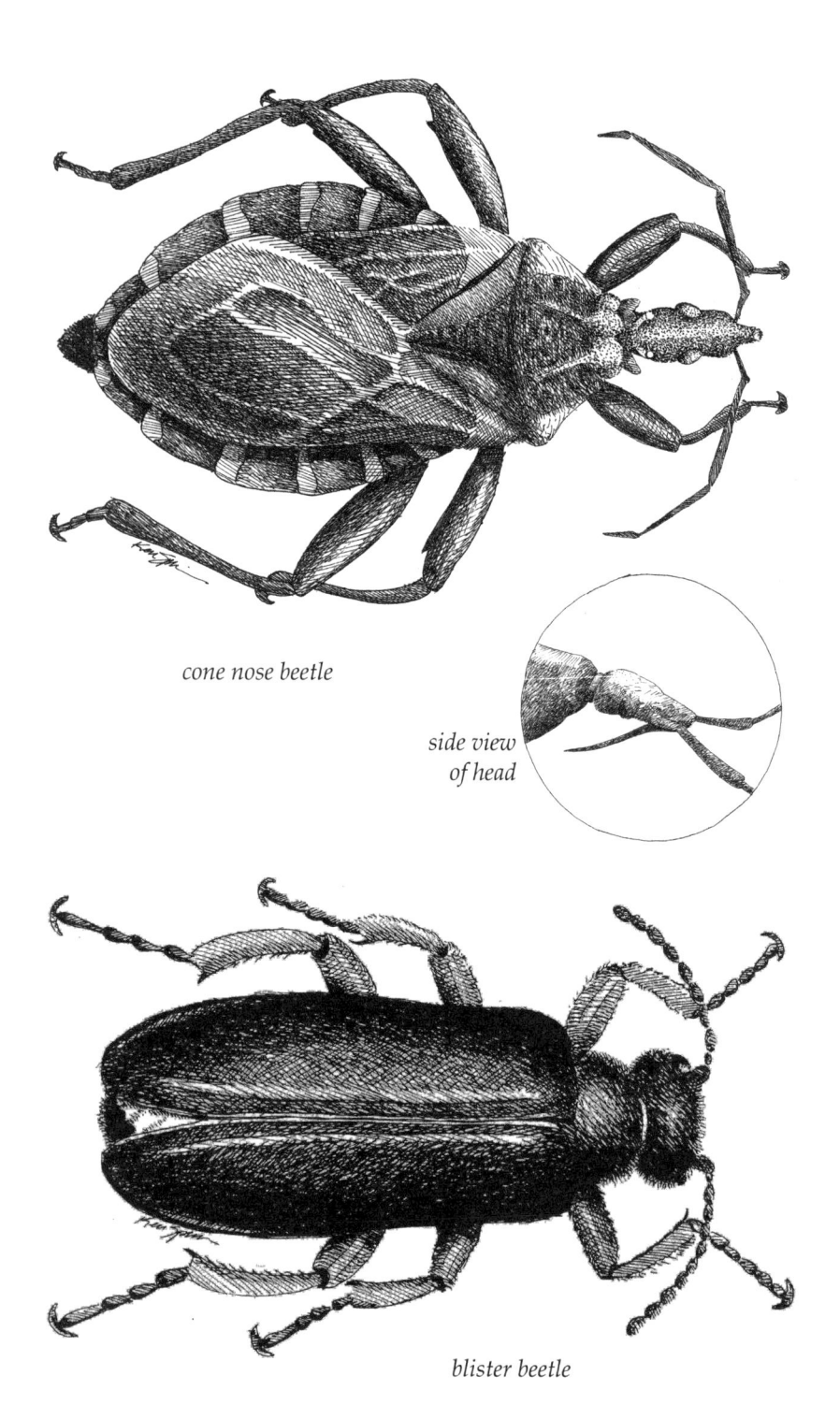

cone nose beetle

side view of head

blister beetle

Kissing Bugs, Cone Nose Beetles, Hualapai Tigers

This insect with various names, same bug, is a generic beetle-looking creature about one-half to three-fourths inch long. These bugs have a raindrop-shaped body; flat back; a round belly that is dark brown, almost black, in color; a skinny neck; and a nearly non-existent head with two big round eyes and a long sucking tube for a mouth. They like to sneak up on people at night and suck their blood, leaving a mound-shaped, feverish red welt about the size of quarter. We use Bigfoot's Bee/Insect Sting Remedy; a tincture of Echinacea, Desert Plantain, or Desert Tobacco; or a Prickly Pear cactus pad. These remedies have worked well for us. There are probably other remedies, too. Purslane would probably be good.

We have read that bites, if untreated, could lead to contracting something like Rocky Mountain fever. Sounds dreadful! Keep in mind that all types of parasites and bites do tax our immune system.

I read somewhere that kissing bugs breed in pack rat nests. I am glad not to be a pack rat. We kill a lot of these bugs in our chicken coop at night in summertime.

Blister Beetles

Blister beetles are slender, cylindrical beetles, from about one-quarter to one inch long, that travel in herds and actually have a noticeable aura of intelligence. We find them eating amaranth, tomatoes, Purslane, and mesquite. If they bite or piss on us, the fluid causes a blister, which will develop into a painful open, wet, ulcerated sore. If not tended to, it seems to get worse. The only remedy we have found is a tincture of Canaigre root, or the root juice, applied to the sore. Canaigre root has a strong astringent quality and is rich in tannic acid.

Walnut tree

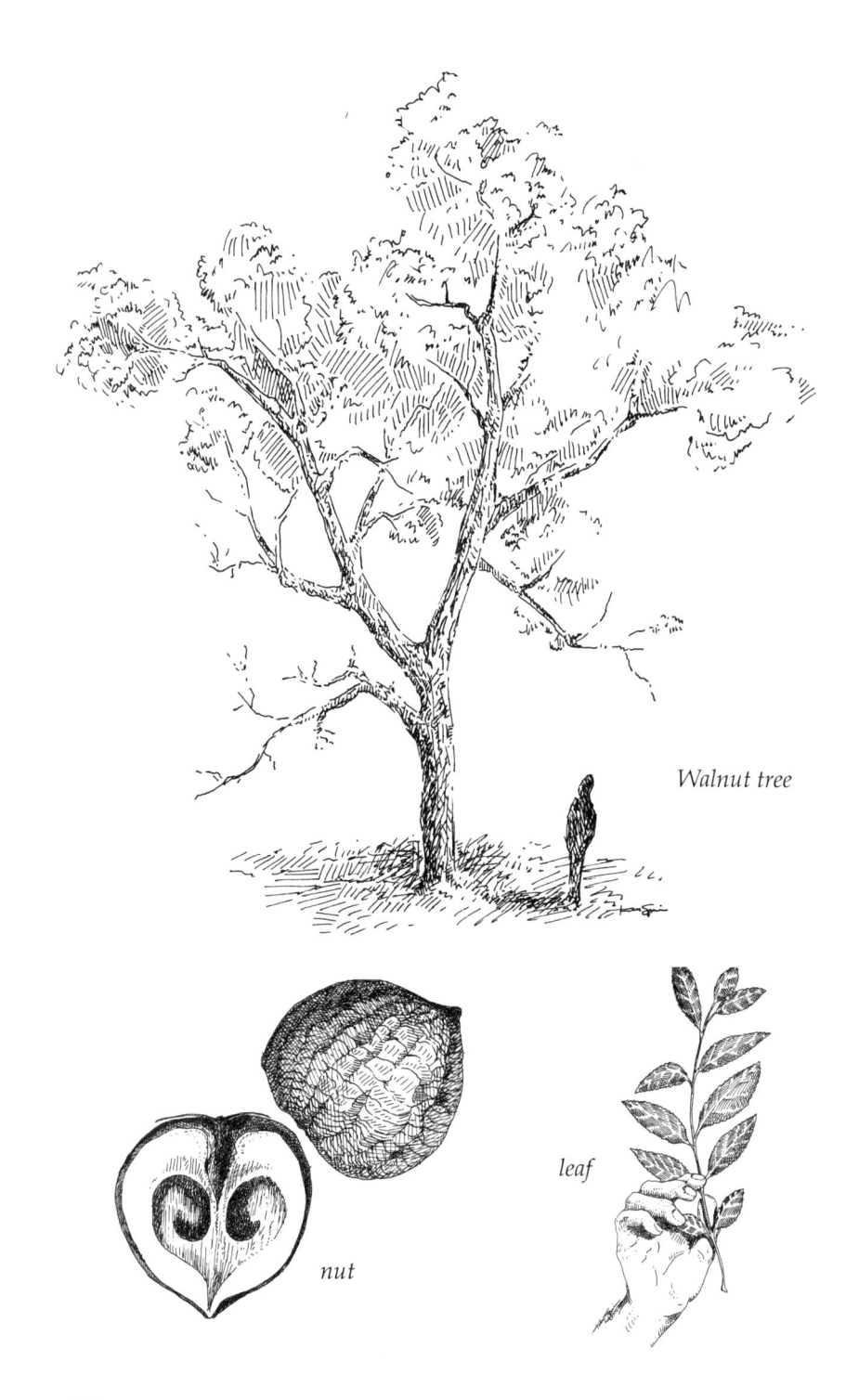

nut

leaf

Gila Monsters

We have had no personal experience with the beady lizard's bite. From our experience with other venomous bites, we would treat it as a snake bite—after peeling the lizard's jaws off the body with a pair of pliers! I've heard that they clamp on and don't let go. I've also heard that holding them under water gets them to let go.

Other Animal Bites

We treat most animal bites the same as a puncture wound and apply a poultice or an antiseptic pine tar salve. For deep bites, we would shoot the remedy down into the holes with a syringe at first to clean them.

Animal bites can get seriously infected rather quickly. Treat them vigorously, don't fool around.

We occasionally get bit or scratched by our farm cats or poultry, and we have noticed that these bites and scratches get rapidly infected. Putting Canaigre tincture on them has brought instant relief. Desert Willow leaf as a tincture or a strong tea (externally) is also a favorite.

Remedies

The best thing I've discovered for this often dangerous type of wound is a poultice of Desert Willow leaves made from the dried and powdered leaves, reconstituted with hot water into a paste. Apply a mass of this material to the wound and bandage it on. Many times any infection will be gone overnight. Leave the poultice on as long as it takes the wound to heal. This method can also be used as a preventive measure against infection of the wound.

Canaigre

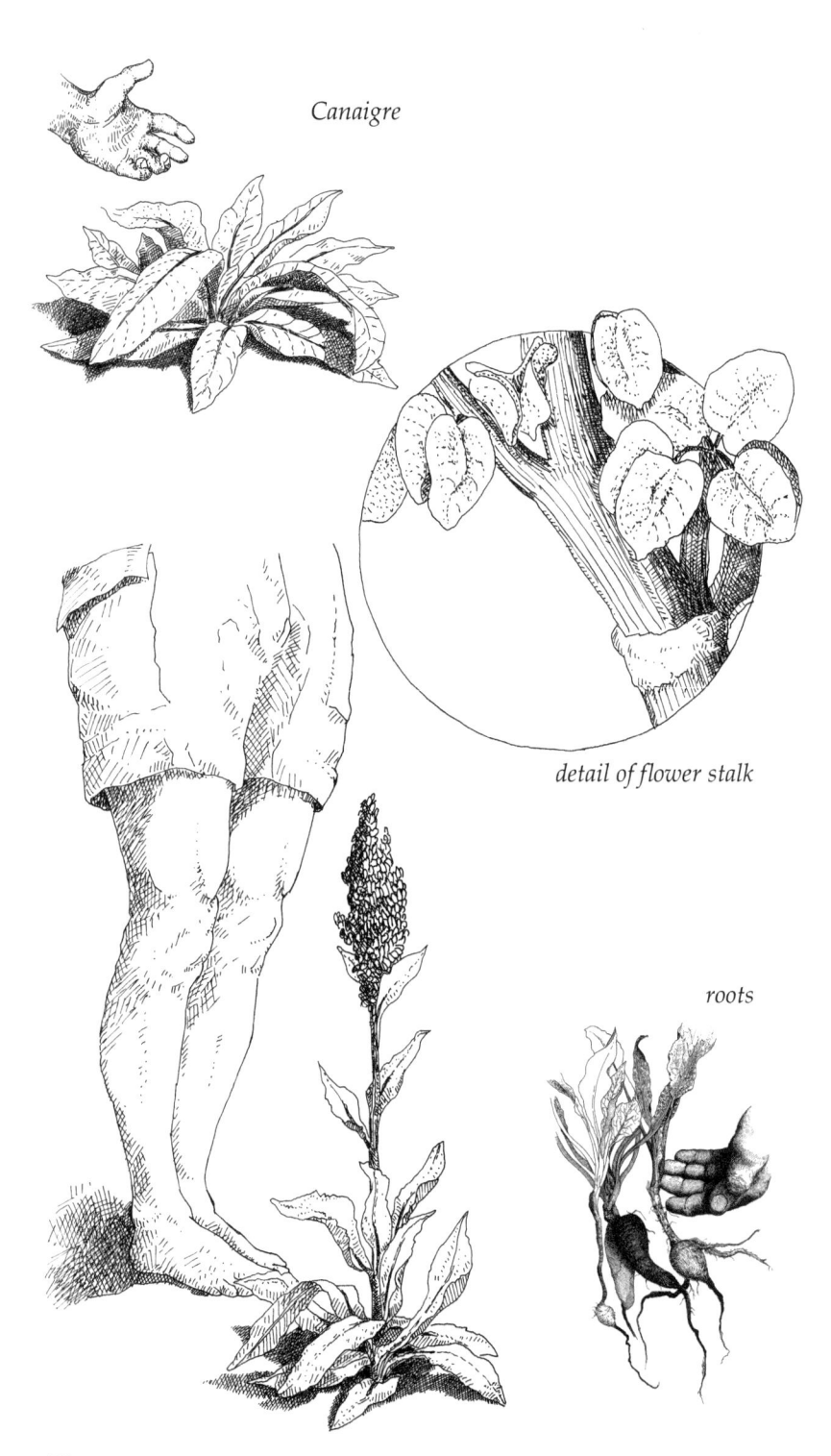

detail of flower stalk

roots

58

Walnut tree bark (tincture) is also among our most trusted remedies for puncture wounds such as animal bites. Some other choices would be the application of a fomentation of Yellow Dock root, Chaparral, Oshá root, Algerita root, Goldenseal, Canaigre root, Echinacea, or Cypress tree cone, all as an alcohol-based tincture (best) or a strong tea. The tincture is best because the alcohol helps the body absorb the herb, and it is usually quicker to get onto the wound. Or, use Bigfoot's All-Purpose Healing Salve.

Rabid Animal Bites

An animal with rabies will have abnormal friendly or vicious behavior, or a wild animal may seem to be tame. It may have a small or large amount of slimy or frothy, thick, lathery saliva. The saliva is usually gray in color and appears just around the edges of the mouth or smeared on the face. It may not be obvious at first glance. The eyes may look dull, dry, or gray. These descriptions depend upon the stage of rabies that the animal is experiencing.

   Infected fleas cause rabies when they bite the animal. Humans acquire rabies through the bite of an infected animal or directly from fleas, or by exposure of a mucous membrane or an open wound to contact with infected saliva. The incubation period ranges from one day to one year; the average is 30 to 50 days. The shortest incubation period is with bites on the head or trunk. After the acute symptoms begin, death is likely to occur within three to ten days.

   When a person is bitten by a rabid animal, the wound becomes red and inflamed and is accompanied by pain and spasms. The person gets depressed and restless. The general restlessness increases to

flower stalk

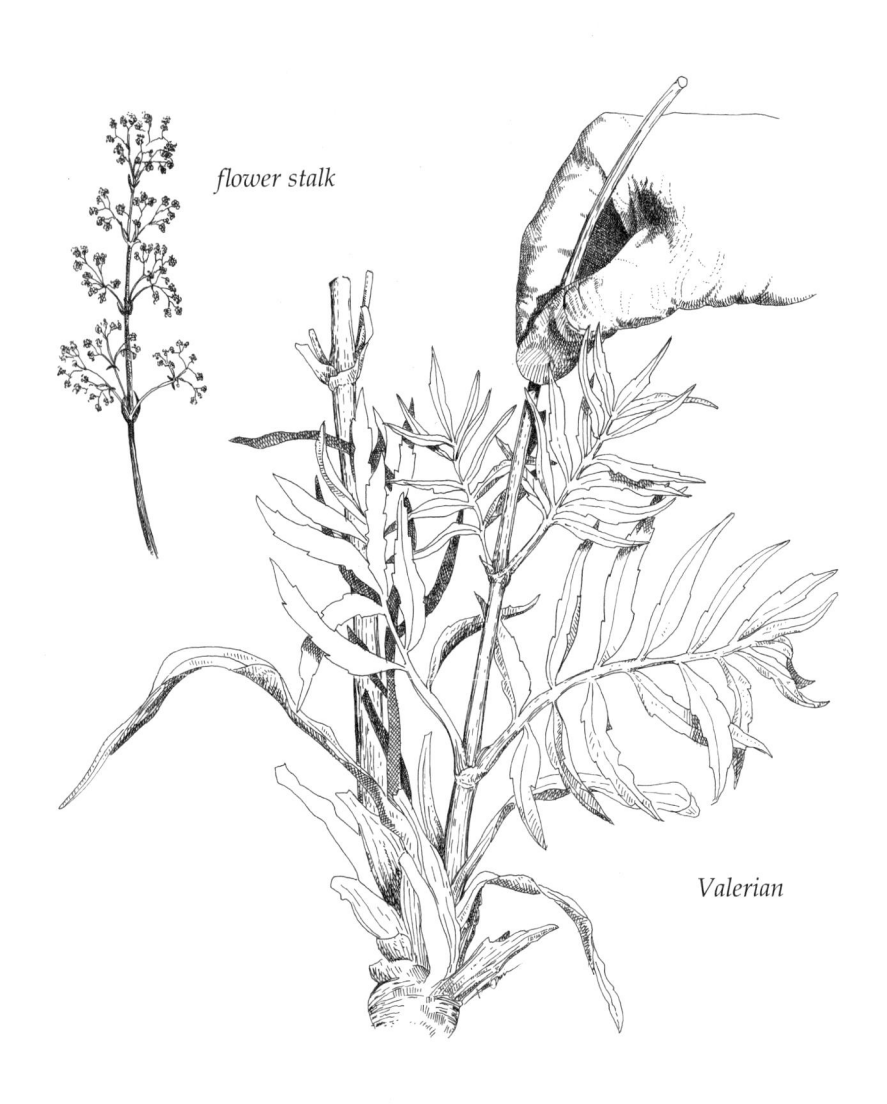

Valerian

uncontrollable excitement. There is a desire to bite something. Possibly there will be difficulty in breathing. The sight of water or shiny objects is distressing; a breeze may bother the person. There will be excessive salivation and difficulty in breathing, as well as excruciating spasms in the neck and throat. The person will be thirsty but repulsed by water, which is why rabies is also called hydrophobia.

Remedies

First, we would flush the wound out with Canaigre root tincture or a tea or tincture of Walnut bark.

Fomentations

Our first choice for treating a rabid animal bite is a fomentation made with a tincture of Walnut bark, Desert Willow leaf, or Yellow Dock root. Fomentations of Canaigre (root tincture or juice), Echinacea (root tincture), Oshá (root tincture), or Wild Iris (tincture) have also worked. Cypress cone tea or tincture is worth trying. It is a miraculous antiseptic.

Herb Teas

Tea made from Common Ash tree root bark, Green Gentian root, Walnut tree bark, Desert Willow bark, Yellow Dock root, or Echinacea root would be good. There are many other herbs that would be helpful; those listed here are the ones that I would presently use and that either grow here or I have on hand.

Steam Bath

If rabies gets to the advanced stages, the most important treatment is to take hot steam baths at 140°F.

A doctor contracted rabies from one of his patients. When it was apparent that he would die from the sickness, he decided to take a steam bath and roast himself to death. To his amazement, the steam bath cured him. This story is from *Back to Eden,* Jethro Kloss's classic herb book.

Poison Ivy

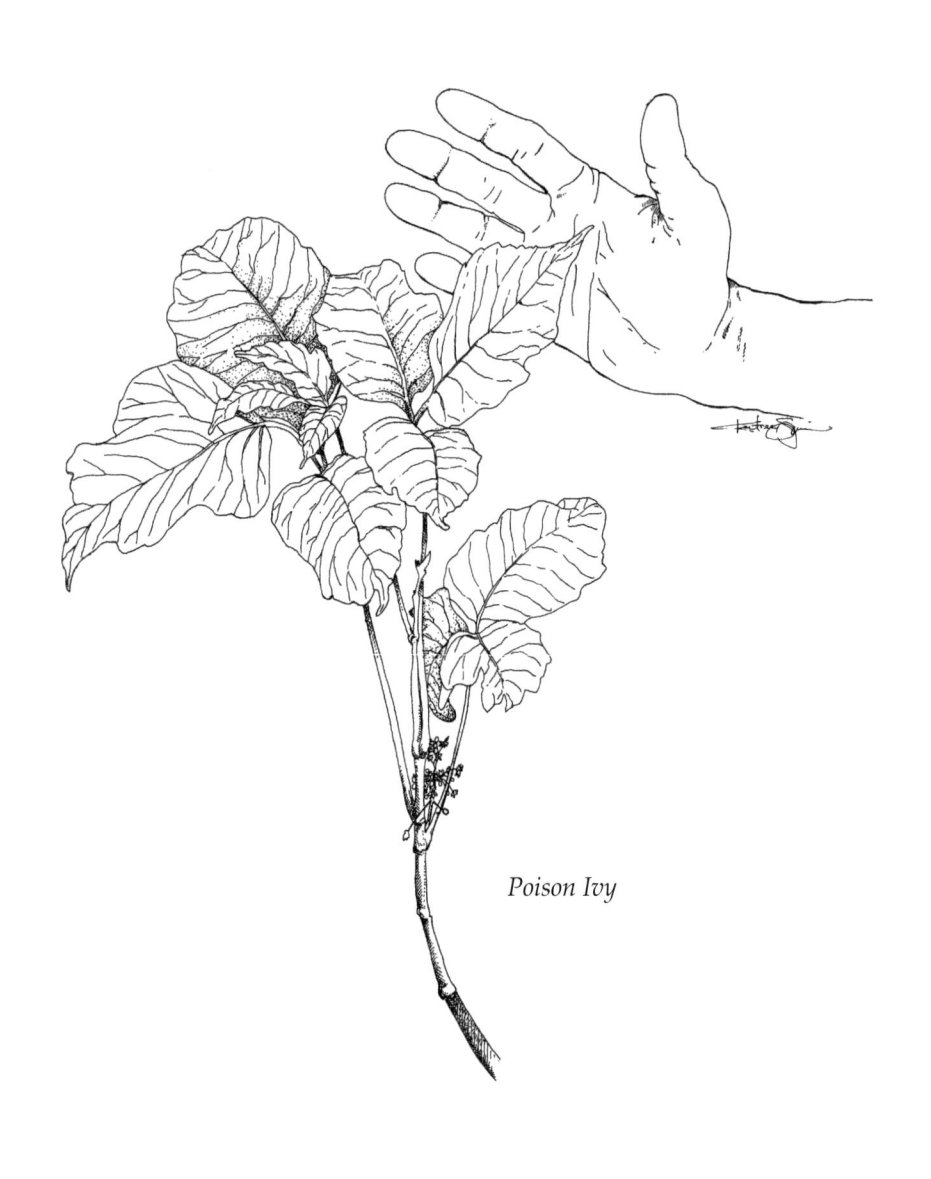

Leaves of three – leave it be!
From berries of white – take flight!
Beans of red will leave you dead!

Poison Ivy

Poison Ivy (*Toxicodendron radicans*) is a plant of the Sumac family, with leaves of three and white berries.

Some people are very allergic to this plant, while others find it to be a useful or even friendly plant. My brother, Charlie, never got an allergic reaction to it, while I did. Some Indian tribes in the Northwest use the vines to make baskets and are not allergic.

One day while out fishing along the Poison Ivy paradise of the Passaic River in New Jersey, I climbed a Poison Ivy–covered tree to retrieve my fishing lure. Then I slipped and fell into the river. That is when I discovered that contact with Poison Ivy can be washed off.

On another fishing adventure, I watched a deer eat nothing but Poison Ivy for half an hour in springtime. Ever since then I eat a few leaves in springtime, and I am about 95% immune to the allergic reaction.

Poison Ivy comes in two different forms. One is a stout, hairy-looking vine that clings to trees. The other grows as thin vines along the ground that put up straight vertical stems 12 to 36 inches high. Both types have similar leaves of three on single stems and clusters of white, peppercorn-sized berries in late summer. The new leaves in springtime are shiny and a mix of bronze and green color. Poison Ivy likes to grow in moist, shady places near streams of water.

Physical contact with any part of the plant, even after the leaves have fallen in autumn and winter, can cause an itching rash. When we are hot and sweaty in summer, we are most vulnerable. Some people can get the rash just from being near the plant at this time.

The most serious reactions come from breathing the smoke of the burning plants. I have heard that people can die from this one. A tea of Western Mugwort has

Wild Grape

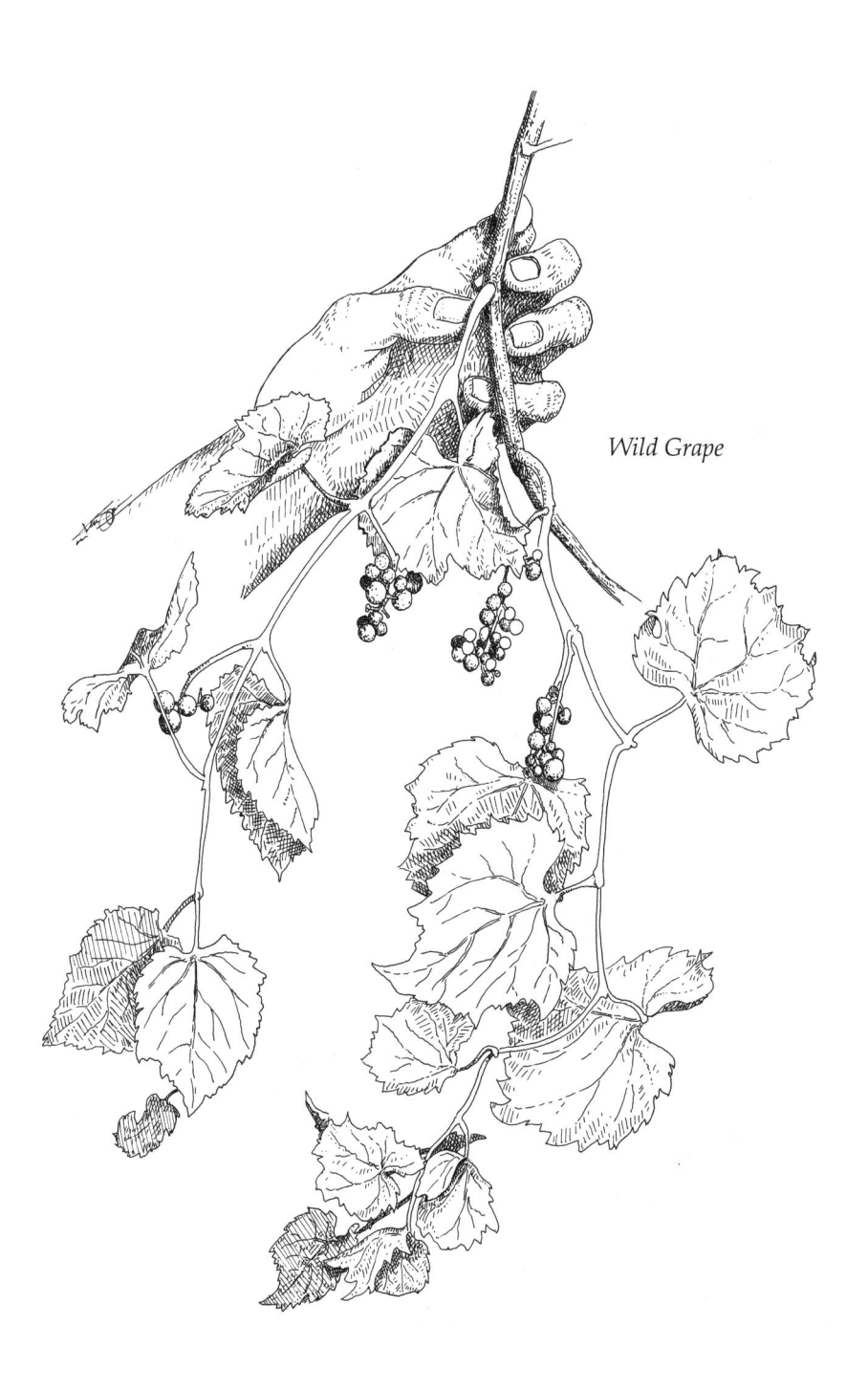

worked well as a remedy for Poison Ivy in the lungs, as well as for external itching.

One springtime I ate quite a lot of Lambsquarter raw in salad and steamed as greens. That summer I was surprised to contract the allergic rash from Poison Ivy several times. Then a friend got it on about 50% of her body (not from me!). In trying to find a remedy for her, we discovered some interesting things. Taking an iron supplement (ferrous sulfate) helped to alleviate the rash. We later learned that eating Lambsquarter depletes iron reserves in our bodies and makes us more allergic to Poison Ivy.

Some of the wild remedies that have worked well for me are rubbing in the fresh juice of Lanceleaf Plantain, Jewel Weed, or Wild Grape leaf; chewing and then rubbing in the leaves of English Lavender or Western Mugwort; and hot fomentations of Yerba Santa or the inner bark (cambium) of Oak, Walnut, Alder, or Sycamore tree.

The Echinacea root tincture method is to scratch the rash until it bleeds. Then apply Echinacea root tincture with cotton balls, with a vengeance! It works.

There are many wonderful remedies for this troublesome rash. Best to get on it right away before the rash has a chance to spread. The two remedies I esteem as being near miraculous are the fresh leaves of Lanceleaf Plantain and English Lavender.

Cold heals the rash, heat aggravates it.

Once, I had a Poison Ivy rash starting on my left arm and happened to walk by an English Lavender plant. I decided to see if it would serve as a remedy. I picked some leaves, chewed them up a bit to express some juice, and rubbed the juicy leaves into the rash. Much to my pleasure, all traces of the rash were gone in an hour. Similar results can be expected from Lanceleaf Plantain used in the same way.

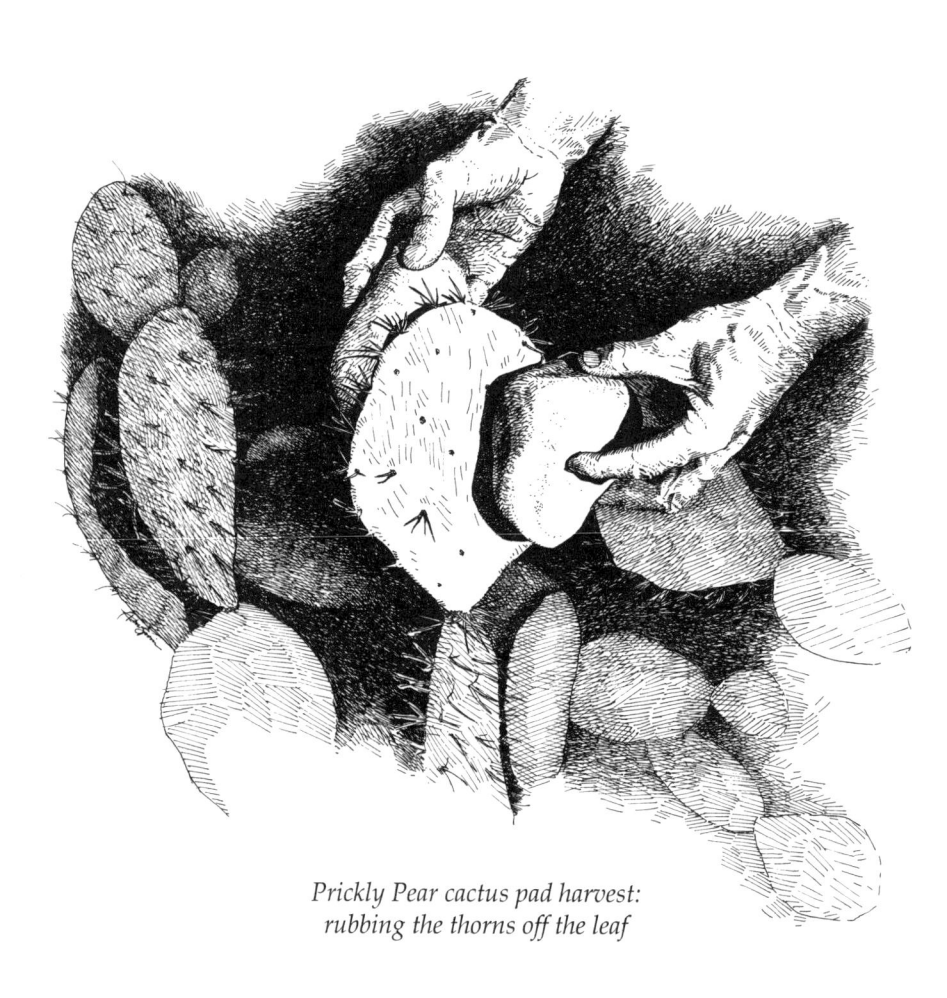

*Prickly Pear cactus pad harvest:
rubbing the thorns off the leaf*

How to Make the Remedies

Poultices

A poultice is a healing bandage that we make by mashing up plant materials and placing this mash on our skin, so the body can use the plant nutrients for healing in the area. Sometimes we use the plant materials intact, such as Datura leaves. We stack these up in a thick pile and apply the stack to the bite or sting.

Keep the poultice in good condition until the healing has taken place. Before the poultice becomes dried out or spoiled, it must be replaced. A poultice may get too hot from absorbing heat from the wound and should then be replaced.

Fresh Plant Poultice

Mash the fresh plant to release its juices. Generally, the larger the poultice (plant mass), the better. The plant mass is held in place with gauze and tape or a cloth bandage and should be kept moist. When using nonpoisonous plants, I sometimes chew them up a little and then place on the wound.

Dried Plant Poultice

Powder the dried herb in a grinder. Sift out the powder from the fibers. It may be stored in this form. To use, mix the powder with hot water, a little at a time, to the consistency of cookie dough, until it does not absorb any more water.

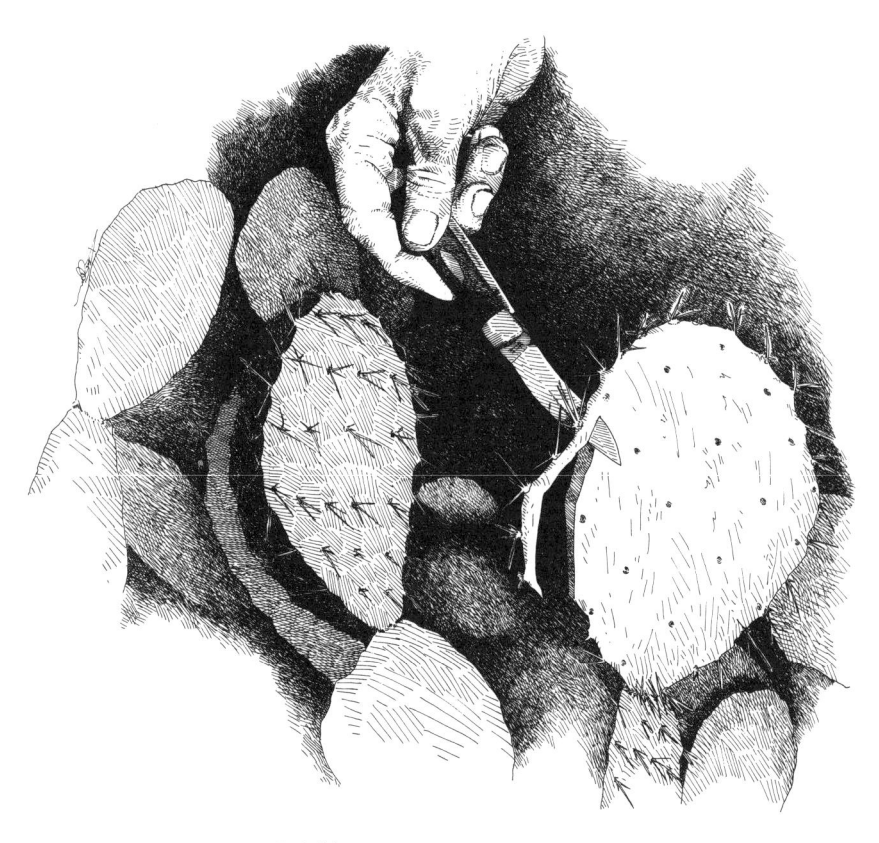

*Prickly Pear cactus pad harvest:
removing the outer edges of the leaf*

Avoid making the poultice material soupy, because you would lose a lot of the plant nutrients in the water. Keep the nutrients in the plant mash.

Allow the mixture to cool before placing on a stung or bitten area. Then apply the mixture to the wound site with gauze and tape or a cloth bandage. The larger the poultice, the better. Flip it over once in a while to keep the bite area cool, or, better, change the poultice now and then to keep it fresh.

Honey Poultice

Saturate the wound with honey. Then place a previously honey-saturated cloth over the wound. Tape on as much additional bandage as necessary to keep the honey from dripping all over the place. A honey bandage is most often used for serious injuries, infections, burns, abrasions, and growing back flesh. Add more honey often; don't let it dry out. We use a bandage so we can move around. If moving around isn't necessary, it is better to just keep the wound saturated with honey and use no covering bandage.

Prickly Pear Poultice

Choose from a healthy-looking cactus the thickest, fattest leaf or pad. To get at the inner flesh, rub the thorns off the flat sides of the leaf with a rough-surfaced rock while supporting the other side with another rock. Next, cut off the outer edges of the cactus pad with a knife. Be certain all the spines and glochids are removed, and cut the leaf free from the cactus. Then slice it through the middle like a hamburger bun, exposing the inner flesh. See the pictures on pages 66, 68, and 70.

Claw the inner flesh with your fingernails to make the surface more juicy. Apply the pad to the afflicted area with its inner side against the skin, and tape or

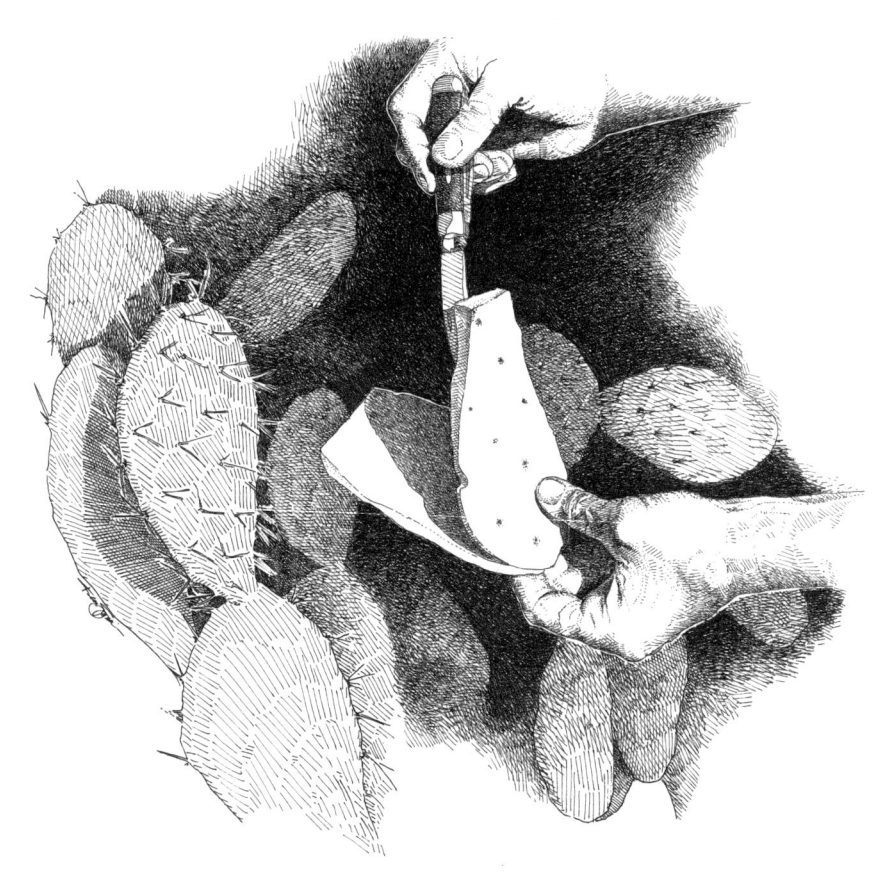

*Prickly Pear cactus pad harvest:
slicing the leaf to expose the inner flesh*

bandage it in place. Sometimes it absorbs so much heat from the wound that it must be changed. It may be necessary to change the pad often. If the pad felt cool and soothing when you put it on and a while later feels hot, itchy, or painful, change it for a fresh one.

Hedgehog Cactus Harvest

Select one of the cactus's "arms" to use. Cut off the top, then peel the cactus like a cucumber, and then cut it off from the base of the plant. Now you can make slices for the poultice. This will require a knife.

Barrel Cactus Poultice Ready-Made for Snake Bite, etc.

An excellent remedy is a ready-made poultice of Barrel cactus. To use it, put eight ounces or more of the cactus mush in a cheesecloth sack to hold the poultice together. Place the poultice over the bite and leave it in place for at least 12 hours. The bite should be healed by then. If not, the poultice can be left on longer.

To prepare the mush, cut out some of the white, juicy pulp from the lower one-third of the Barrel cactus, the area characterized by black needles. Run it through a clean meat grinder to achieve the consistency of raw hamburger. Don't lose any juice.

To preserve the remedy, mix in approximately one-third teaspoon of vitamin C crystals per eight ounces of pulp. Or you can use one tablespoon of Lemonade bush berries. Place the ground pulp in a clean eight-ounce wide-mouth canning jar, leaving a half inch of head room. Place the lid on loosely.

Store in a cool, dark place for seven days so that it will reach its greatest potency. Avoid freezing, which may cause spoilage.

milky sap from stem

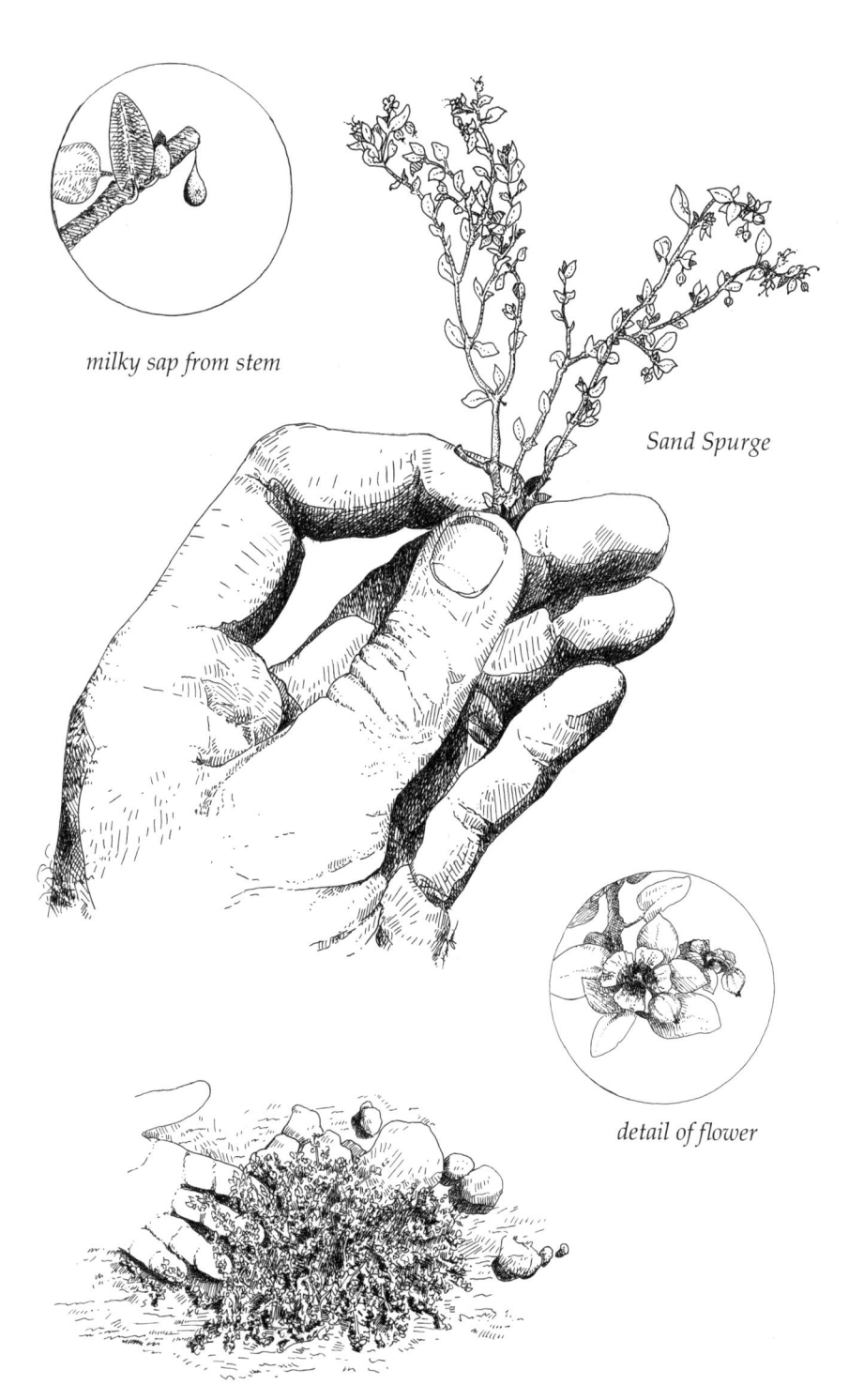

Sand Spurge

detail of flower

Within a three-day period the preparation may overflow its container. After this happens you can tighten the lid. After it sits for 60 days without any problem it probably will last a year and can travel in your backpack. Avoid getting it in direct sunlight. I suspect that it loses some potency with age.

The person who taught me this remedy said it would completely heal a fresh bite in less than three hours.

Fresh Barrel Cactus Poultice

To make a Barrel cactus poultice fresh on the spot in the "wild," mash the cactus flesh between rocks or grind it up somehow. Apply about a 12-ounce (or more) poultice to the bite area. You'll find it quite soothing and very effective. Grinding it up or mashing the cactus flesh makes its juice and nutrients more available than just a firm chunk of cactus flesh.

Sand Spurge Milk

Break off a Sand Spurge stem and a milky-white droplet of sap should appear. Place this droplet on the bite. Repeat this about 20 times or so until the bite is well covered with sap. The plant will not always have available sap, depending on the time of year.

Fomentations

A fomentation is a strong herb tea, soaked into a cloth or cotton wadding and placed on the afflicted area. A fomentation is most often used when the plant material is too gnarly (such as woody roots and tree bark) to place on the skin or wound. See instructions below for making tea.

Four Wing Salt Bush

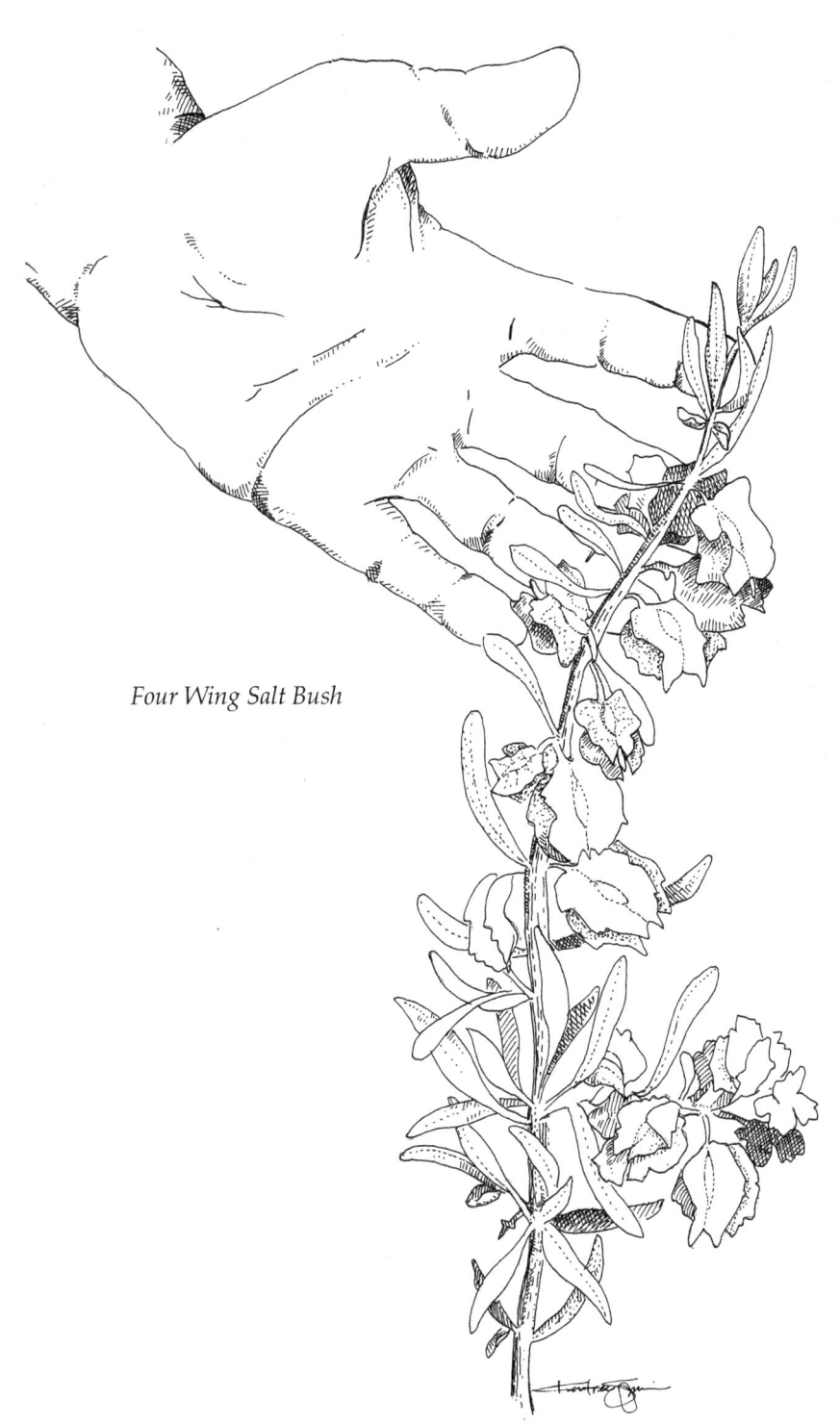

Tincture Fomentation

Place a dry mass of cotton wadding or cloth over the afflicted area. Tape or bandage it on. Then squirt the tincture in to saturate the cotton. Keep it moist. If you wet the cotton first, too often the tape will not stick to the wet skin. If you don't have wadding or cloth, use mud instead (a mud poultice).

Herb Teas

A tea results from extracting the nutrients from a plant substance into water. In general, we steep (soak in hot water) leaves and flowers, and we simmer roots, leathery leaves, and barks for 15 to 30 minutes. (A simmered tea is called a decoction.) Keep a lid on the pot while steeping or simmering so as not to lose the herbal essence into the air.

Some herbs are stronger than others. The general rule to find what strength works for you is to start with one teaspoon of herb to a cup of hot water. If it brews up too strong, then add water until it is palatable.

Be sure you know how much of an herb to take at one time, as some herbs can have toxic or discomforting effects if used in excessive doses. Indiscriminate combinations are not wise. Sometimes they work real well and sometimes they don't. Most often the wisest choice is a single herb, carefully selected for its purpose. The more experience we gain with practice, the more accurate will be our intuition. Pay attention to how you feel while drinking an herb tea. If a discomforting effect develops, then quit drinking the tea, or drink less. If it makes you feel better, then maybe take more.

To prepare a tea for a fomentation, make it about three to ten times stronger than you would for drinking.

When using bark, we use the inner cambium layer

Camphor weed

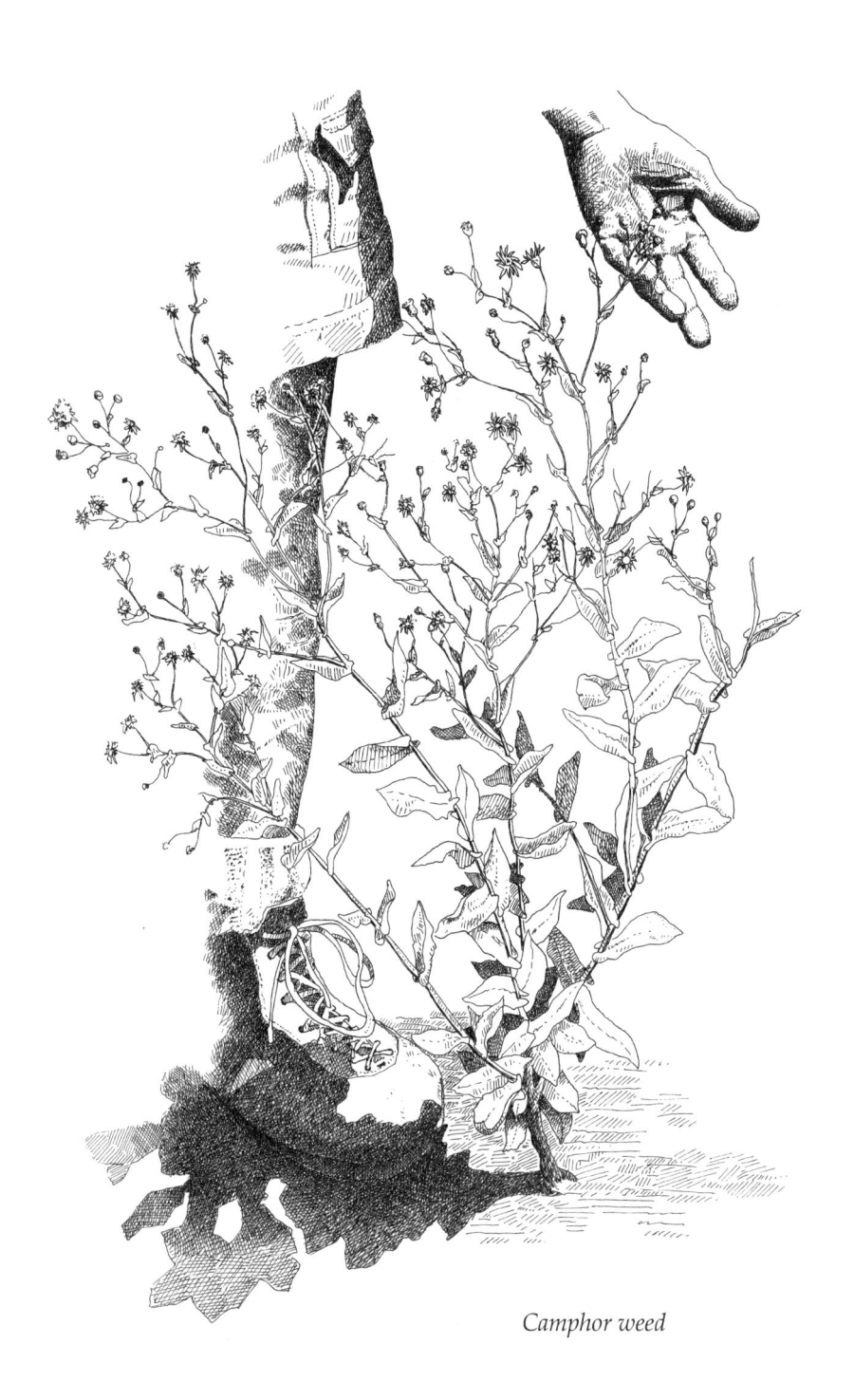

(growth layer), not the outer bark. If the outer protective layer of bark is thin and smooth like a skin (like Aspen bark), leave it attached to the cambium. If it is thick and scaly (like old Oak bark), shave it off the inner bark.

Canaigre Root Juice

To make this magical astringent antiseptic, run the fresh roots of Canaigre through a carrot juicer. It may then be applied. To preserve it for later use, let the juice sit for about a month in a tall jar, until it separates. The pure, clear black liquid is what we want. You can figure out how to separate it out. This black liquid is fungus-static and bacterial-static and therefore will not spoil if kept in a cool, dark place in a glass container for up to a year.

Another way to use Canagrie is to slice the roots, dry them, and powder them, and then make a tincture or fomentation.

Urine Therapy

Urine therapy is the healing use of one's own urine, either externally or internally. It is believed by those who use their own urine for healing themselves that the body makes antibodies that come out in the urine—a homeopathic remedy. Therefore, when using urine for a remedy, collect it after you have been bitten or stung.

Imagine three portions of the released urine: the first, middle, and last. Only collect the middle portion to use for the remedy. From this, drink about one to two ounces.

I personally haven't had enough experience with this method to make a worthy comment on it. However, it does have some firm believers.

Camphor weed flower detail

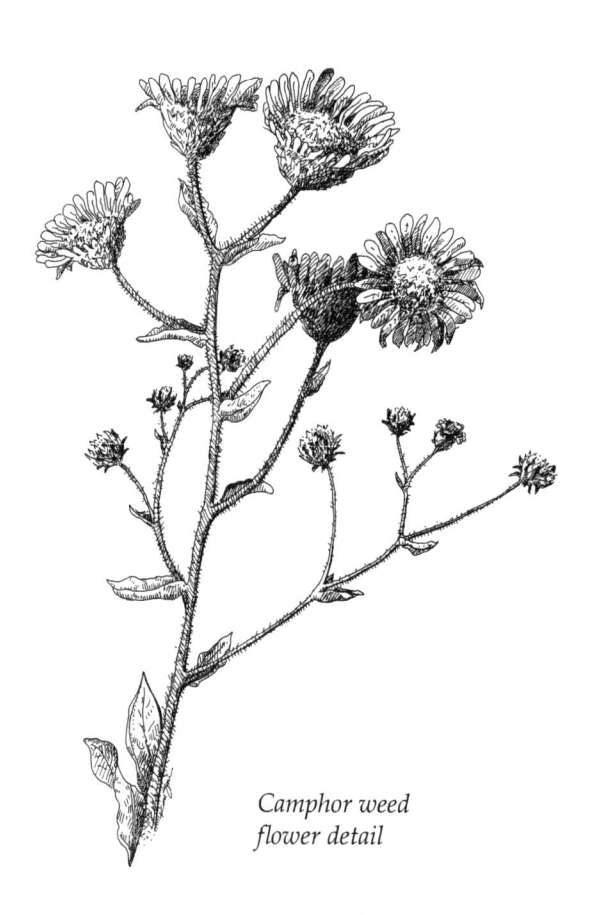

Reevis Mountain School of Self-Reliance

Reevis Mountain School was founded and created by Peter "Bigfoot" Busnack, a man of many occupations, and Phoenix-based attorney John "Azimuth" Goodson. These men teamed up in 1979 to fulfill Peter's lifelong dream of using his many practical skills and broad experiences to create a homestead in the wilderness and live there. Many others joined in to be of assistance in this endeavor and to experience wilderness living.

It soon became evident that the skills demonstrated here at Reevis and the results of our labors were of great value to many people who came here to learn. Thus the school was born to fill an expressed need, offering classes in outdoor survival and self-reliance skills, with a focus on awareness and expanding consciousness, plant identification, natural healing, self-discovery, meditation, stone masonry, land navigation, organic gardening, and community living. Peter and his wife, Patricia, are directors of the school.

Many of our students feel this high-speed, high-tech world may one day collapse in on itself and that the skills and understandings taught here at Reevis will be vital; others have simply found city life to be meaningless. They want to know how to feed themselves from nature, and how to heal illness and injury without going to a medical doctor (who is expensive to consult, may not be available when needed, and often is at a loss to heal conditions that would respond well to simple natural remedies). Reevis's students want to know who are we? Is this all there is?

Why are we here? Awareness of the answers to these questions provides a great feeling of security and serenity.

For further information about RMS and our classes and products, please write Reevis Mountain School, 7448 S. J-B Ranch Rd., Roosevelt, AZ 85545, or visit www.reevismountain.org.

Live what you love and follow a path of joy.

God Bless You,

Peter Bigfoot